101
Foot Care
Tips
for
People
with
Diabetes

Jessie H. Ahroni, PhD, ARNP, CDE

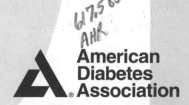

American
Diabetes
Association

Book Acquisitions	Robert J. Anthony
Editor	Sherrye Landrum
Production Director	Carolyn R. Segree
Production Coordinator	Peggy M. Rote
Composition	Harlowe Typography, Inc.
Cover Design	Wickham & Associates, Inc.
Printer	Transcontinental Printing Inc.

Printed in Canada

1 3 5 7 9 10 8 6 4 2

The suggestions and information contained in this publication are generally consistent with the *Clinical Practice Recommendations* and other policies of the American Diabetes Association, but they do not represent the policy or position of the Association or any of its boards or committees. Reasonable steps have been taken to ensure the accuracy of the information presented. However, the American Diabetes Association cannot ensure the safety or efficacy of any product or service described in this publication. Individuals are advised to consult a physician or other appropriate health care professional before undertaking any diet or exercise program or taking any medication referred to in this publication. Professionals must use and apply their own professional judgment, experience, and training and should not rely solely on the information contained in this publication before prescribing any diet, exercise, or medication. The American Diabetes Association— its officers, directors, employees, volunteers, and members—assumes no responsibility or liability for personal or other injury, loss, or damage that may result from the suggestions or information in this publication.

ADA titles may be purchased for business or promotional use or for special sales. For information, please write to Lee Romano Sequeira, Special Sales & Promotions, at the address below.

American Diabetes Association
1701 North Beauregard Street
Alexandria, Virginia 22311

Library of Congress Cataloging-in-Publication Data

Ahroni, Jessie H., 1948–
    101 foot care tips for people with diabetes / Jessie H. Ahroni.
      p. cm.
    Includes index.
    ISBN 1-58040-040-X (pbk. : acid-free paper)
      1. Foot—Diseases—Popular works. 2. Diabetes—Complications. 3. Self-care, Health. I.
    Title: One hundred one foot care tips for people with diabetes.

RC951.A38 2000
617.5'85—dc21   99-055685

101 FOOT CARE TIPS FOR PEOPLE WITH DIABETES

▼

TABLE OF CONTENTS

PREFACE

During the last few years, the treatment of diabetes has changed. As well as new medications and testing devices, there is an increased emphasis on keeping blood sugar levels as close to normal as possible. These improvements in diabetes treatment will permit many people with diabetes to avoid or delay the onset of diabetic foot complications. However, there are many others who have lived with diabetes for a long time before good blood sugar control was possible or the importance of it was clearly understood. This book is dedicated to all the people who have been my patients and research subjects over the years. I have learned more from them than from any formal educational experience. I have learned about true courage and what real strength is all about. These people get up every morning of their lives and go out and take on the world, but they do it with the burden of diabetes—a burden that few people without the disease can imagine. I honor and admire them, and sincerely appreciate the opportunity to share this collection of their suggestions and experiences with other people who have diabetes. I hope that many of these tips will apply to you and help you care for your feet and avoid the foot complications that are too often associated with diabetes.

Chapter 1
GENERAL TIPS

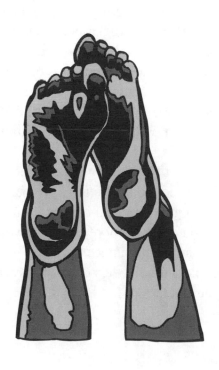

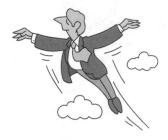

*W*hy is it important for me to take
special care of my feet?

▼
TIP:

If you want to be active and independent all of your life—whether or not you have diabetes—you need to have healthy feet. Most people take their feet for granted, but people with diabetes really cannot do that. You are challenged by two complications of diabetes that can affect the nerves and blood vessels of the feet—diabetic nerve damage and poor circulation. These complications make it easier for you to get a foot ulcer that will not heal. Nonhealing ulcers lead to amputation, which will severely limit what you can do for yourself.

The good news is that by taking good care of your feet, you can often prevent diabetic foot complications. If you take care of your feet every day and get good medical care as soon as you even suspect you might need it, you're much more likely to avoid getting the infections that make amputation necessary. In fact, at least 50% of amputations in people with diabetes could be prevented this way. You can protect your feet.

*W*hat foot problems do people with diabetes experience?

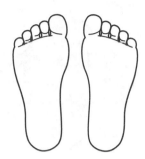

▼
TIP:

People with diabetes have the same foot problems that people without diabetes experience—corns, calluses, bunions, ingrown toenails, arthritis, and broken bones. However, these ordinary foot problems can be more serious in people with diabetes if they also have diabetic nerve disease or poor circulation.

People with diabetic nerve damage cannot feel with their feet normally, so they may not notice an injury, sores, or even high-pressure areas on their feet. They may continue to walk on an injury or high-pressure spot that would cause pain in a person without nerve damage. This continued walking might cause a wound or ulcer. Once the skin is broken, the ulcer can become infected. The blood supply carries oxygen, white blood cells that attack bacteria, and healing nutrients to wounds. It also carries any antibiotics that you take. But if you don't have enough blood supply to the foot, an ulcer can be difficult or impossible to heal. If not treated, some of these foot infections will lead to amputation.

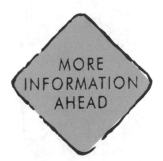

MORE
INFORMATION
AHEAD

A m I more likely to get an infection just because I have diabetes?

▼
TIP:

Yes. People with diabetes who have high blood sugars most of the time are more likely to develop infections than people with normal blood sugars. High blood sugars can interfere with your body's natural defense systems so infections are harder to heal, too.

Healthy skin is your main defense against infection, and diabetes can make your skin dry and more susceptible to cracking. Once the skin is broken, germs can enter. Fungal diseases that appear in folds of skin and on your feet need sugar and moisture to grow, and they like high blood glucose levels. The damage they do to your skin can allow infection to begin.

How common are diabetic foot problems?

▼
TIP:

The short answer is way too common. About half of the people who have diabetes for 10 years will have some degree of nerve damage. The older you are and the longer you have had diabetes, the more likely you are to have nerve damage—but not everybody gets it. Recent studies show that people who maintain good blood sugar control are less likely to develop nerve damage or poor blood circulation.

It is estimated that 15–25% of people with diabetes will have a foot ulcer at least once. About 70% of these ulcers will heal with good basic foot care. Up to 10% of people with diabetes will have an amputation at some time in their lives. Toe and partial foot amputations are the most common, followed by below-the-knee amputations. Amputation rates are greater with increasing age, in males compared with females, and among African Americans and Hispanic Americans. Experts believe that at least half of these amputations could be prevented by good blood sugar control, better preventive foot care, and better care of foot ulcers.

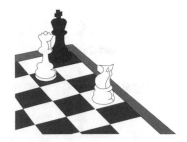

*W*ho is at greatest risk for diabetic
foot problems?

▼
TIP:

The people most at risk have diabetic nerve damage and poor
circulation; have limited joint mobility, deformity, or thick nails;
have already had a foot ulcer or amputation; or have other
complications of diabetes, such as eye disease (retinopathy) or
kidney disease (nephropathy). Once you have a foot ulcer or
amputation, you are likely to get another one. This is because you
have serious damage to the nerves and blood vessels of your feet,
not because you do not take care of your feet. Most people with
diabetes who have had foot problems take better than average care
of their feet, but good foot care alone may not be enough to prevent
foot problems once they are already established.

Newly diagnosed young people with type 1 diabetes who do not
have other complications of diabetes or other foot problems have
little risk. The American Diabetes Association (ADA) recommends
that annual foot risk screening begin 5 years after the diagnosis of
diabetes, but it is never too early to develop good foot care habits.

Older people who are recently diagnosed with type 2 diabetes
may actually have had diabetes for years before they find out about
it and already have complications. If you have type 2 diabetes, start
good foot care right away.

The thought of complications scares me. Why can't I just ignore this until later?

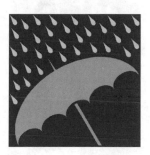

▼
TIP:

Because there are things that you can do right now to lower your risk and prevent the complications of diabetes. Adjusting your food, physical activity, and medications to control your blood sugar may help you avoid or delay complications. Taking good care of your feet will help you keep them. Ignoring your diabetes won't do you any good and is likely to be harmful.

All of us have fears of growing old or disabled. It is normal and appropriate to express these emotions. The challenge is to choose to live well every day. Give yourself the best chance to remain fully functional and independent throughout your life.

Deciding to ignore diabetes and its complications does not stop them or make them go away. Learning about diabetes and your body gives you the power to take charge and direct the outcome so you can live life without fear.

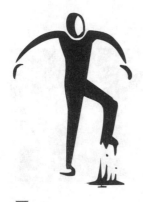

*W*hat can I do to prevent diabetic foot
problems?

▼
TIP:

- Look at and touch your feet every day: tops, bottoms, backs, sides, and between the toes. Get prompt medical attention for any problems.
- Keep your feet clean and dry.
- Cut or file toenails with the shape of the toe, smoothing all sharp edges.
- Moisturize dry skin with a good lotion.
- Avoid injury to your feet. Have corns, calluses, or ingrown toe-nails treated by a professional.
- Wear well-fitting socks, without a thick toe seam, made of a material that wicks moisture away from the skin, such as an acrylic and cotton or wool blend.
- Wear well-fitting soft leather or fabric shoes, such as running shoes. Wear house shoes at home.
- Check shoes daily for cracks, pebbles, or other things that might damage your feet.
- Get your blood glucose under control.
- Have surgery to fix deformities such as bunions and hammertoes.

Does my weight affect my feet?

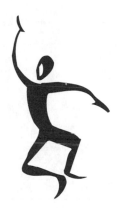

▼
TIP:

Absolutely. This is just common sense. The more we weigh the more stress is transmitted through our knees, ankles, and feet. Many people with foot pain can get relief just by losing weight. Heel pain is one example of a pain that is often weight related. Arthritis pain in the knees and feet is frequently worse in people who are overweight.

People who are obese have a different gait from those who are not. Their feet are placed wider than normal because their thighs hold the legs outward. This places the body weight more towards the inner part of the foot, changing the mechanics of walking completely. There is increased stress on the tendons, ligaments, and joints of the feet.

If you have diabetic neuropathy, your weight is even more important. The stress of additional pounds on numb feet increases the likelihood of your developing ulcers and Charcot deformities.

If you become pregnant, your feet may change shape and size during the pregnancy and for about 6 months after the baby is born. Sometimes they remain permanently larger. Be aware of this and try to wear comfortable, supportive shoes, such as running shoes. High heels are not really a good idea for anyone, but especially not for a pregnant woman.

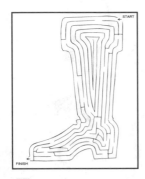

*W*hat does blood sugar control have to do with feet?

TIP:

If you control your blood sugar, you increase your chances of not getting diabetes complications. If you already have complications, you may keep them from getting worse or slow down their progression. With good blood sugar control, you are less likely to develop nerve damage or poor circulation, and you'll heal faster.

Results from the two largest studies of blood sugar control, the Diabetes Control and Complications Trial (DCCT) and the United Kingdom Prospective Diabetes Study (UKPDS), support this. The DCCT studied 1,400 people with type 1 diabetes. Half of the people received "conventional" care (1–2 insulin injections a day), and the other half received "intensive" care (as many injections as needed to keep blood sugar close to the normal range). Patients with near normal blood sugar levels had a 40–70% reduction in the complications of diabetes. This improvement was gained regardless of the patient's age, sex, or length of time they'd had diabetes.

The UKPDS studied the effects of near normal blood sugar levels in 5,200 people with type 2 diabetes by placing them in conventional (diet and exercise) or intensive (oral medications or insulin) care groups. The results were dramatic and showed the same strong benefits of near normal blood sugar levels in preventing or slowing down diabetes complications.

*W*hich health care providers should help
me take care of my feet?

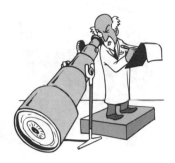

▼
TIP:

The first person to ask about taking care of your feet is your podiatrist or foot care specialist. If you need a referral, ask your primary care or diabetes care provider. At some point, you should see a diabetes educator, usually a nurse, physician's assistant, dietitian, pharmacist, or other health care professional, to learn how to take care of your feet. Sometimes physical therapists are trained to help people with diabetic foot problems. Any of these health professionals may be a certified diabetes educator (CDE) and can help you learn about diabetes and proper care of your feet.

Podiatrists are specially trained to take care of feet and can help you with everything from routine care to foot surgery. Orthopedic surgeons specialize in bone surgery, and some specialize in surgery of the foot and ankle. Vascular surgeons specialize in surgery on the blood vessels, and some specialize in surgery on the blood vessels of the legs and feet. They can help restore circulation to the feet. You would be more likely to see a surgeon if you have problems with an ulcer that won't heal.

Pedorthists are professional shoe fitters who make and fit shoes and insoles for people with foot problems. They can be of great assistance to you, especially if you have lost feeling in your feet.

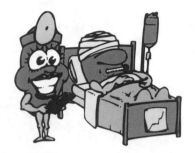

*D*o I need to see a podiatrist or an orthopedic surgeon?

▼
TIP:

Ask your health care provider. You can see a podiatrist for routine foot care if you cannot see well or reach your feet. Podiatrists are doctors of podiatric medicine (DPM), and in most states, diagnose and treat conditions of the feet. They perform routine foot care, such as toenail trimming, callus removal, treatment for ingrown toenails, and perform foot surgery on bones and soft tissue, such as bunion or hammertoe surgery. They can study how your feet and legs work when you move and walk (biomechanics). They can pinpoint bones that are out of place and that put unusual pressure on the skin of your feet. They can design arch supports to help your feet work normally and order special footwear if you need it.

Orthopedic surgeons are medical doctors (MD) who perform surgery on the bones. Some specialize in foot and ankle problems. Orthopedic surgeons do not usually provide routine services like toenail trimming and removing ingrown toenails. They may perform foot surgery. They too can order arch supports and special footwear if you need it.

If you want to find a board-certified podiatrist or orthopedic doctor, check the Resources section.

H̲ow often should I have a doctor take care of my feet?

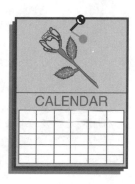

▼
TIP:

Have your feet checked at least once a year, usually at a regular visit. Your health care provider will look for any changes in shape (deformity) that change the way you walk and bear weight on the foot. He'll also check for loss of feeling by pressing a thin plastic wire called a monofilament against the soles of your feet or by holding a vibrating tuning fork against the base of your big toe. The provider will also check your circulation and examine the skin, especially between your toes and under metatarsal heads (bones in the ball of your foot.)

If you can't examine your own feet or if you have foot problems or nerve damage, have your feet checked more often, probably at every visit.

The following are warning signs to have your feet checked:

- Redness, swelling, or increased warmth
- A change in the size or shape of the foot or ankle
- Pain in the legs at rest or while walking
- Open sores with or without drainage, no matter how small
- Nonhealing wounds
- Ingrown toenails
- Corns or calluses with skin discoloration
- Unexplained high blood sugar levels

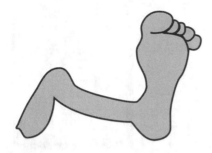

My doctor is busy. How do I get him or her to check my feet?

▼
TIP:

Take off your shoes and socks. If you have trouble doing this, ask the doctor's nurse or assistant to help you. Studies have shown that health care professionals are much more likely to examine the feet of a person with diabetes if the shoes and socks have already been removed when the health care provider comes into the examining room.

Another way to get your feet examined is to ask. Most health care professionals will readily check your feet whenever they are asked.

Finally, if you do not feel that you are getting enough attention to your feet through the regular medical care system, you could go to a podiatrist or orthopedic doctor who specializes in taking care of feet.

I *cannot see my feet very well. How can I take care of them?*

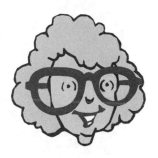

▼
TIP:

S it down and pull your foot up on your knee or rest your foot on a footstool to get it closer to your eyes. Wear your glasses if you need to, and pick a place with good lighting. Use a mirror or magnifying mirror to examine the bottom of your feet. Medical supply stores and large drugstores have mirrors with long handles.

Be sure to run your hands over your feet. People with poor vision can learn what their feet feel like and can pick up changes in their feet by feeling them. If none of these suggestions works and a podiatrist is not available, you might ask a friend or family member for help or get a professional pedicure at a beauty shop.

Do not cut your toenails or do any kind of corn or callus removal if you cannot see well. Your health care provider, a nurse, or assistant, or a home care nurse may be able to help you with foot care. In some communities, foot care is available at senior centers. Another option is to see a professional who specializes in taking care of feet such as a podiatrist.

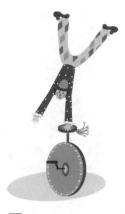

I cannot reach my feet very well. How can I
take care of them?

▼

TIP:

Get a bath bench for your shower or tub in a drugstore or
medical supply store. Have grab bars installed in your shower
or tub. Get a long-handled bath brush or sponge on a handle, so you
can wash your feet while sitting down or holding onto the grab bar.
Rinse your feet before you stand up because soapy feet are slippery.

You can leave one end of the towel on the floor and rub your foot
over the towel to dry it. Dry as well as you can between the toes.
You can also use the sponge on a handle to apply lotion to your feet,
but you need two sponges: one for bathing and one for lotion. Keep
the lotion sponge in a plastic bag.

Most people who have trouble reaching their feet wear slip-on
shoes or shoes with Velcro™ fasteners. You can also try elastic
laces, found in shoe repair shops. A long-handled shoehorn also
comes in handy, as does a "sock-puller."

You might ask for a referral to an occupational therapist. An
occupational therapist can help you find and use devices like sock-
pullers and long-handled shoehorns. If flexibility is part of your
problem, ask for help learning stretching exercises or yoga postures.

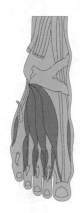

*W*hat changes in the foot are due to
normal aging?

▼
TIP:

Changes can occur in our hardworking feet as we age, especially
joint diseases like arthritis. Bones can shift out of position,
rubbing against shoes and causing pain and the protective buildup of
calluses or corns. We lose some of the fat pad that cushions the ball
of the foot—and people with diabetes may lose it all—causing a
callus to grow as a way to relieve the sharp pressure of bones on the
soles of our feet. This and other changes can make us unsteady, and
our gait or walking pattern may change. Our feet tend to get longer,
wider, and flatter, which affects how our shoes fit.

You can offset some of the effects of aging. Always wear shoes
that fit well. Sometimes changes in the shape of your feet occur so
gradually that you do not notice how poorly your shoes fit, especially
if you have nerve damage and cannot feel your feet. Don't wear
shoes that you have saved for years for special occasions.

An unsteady gait can be a sign of another type of medical
problem, so talk to your provider about it. It may just be time to get
a cane. Your provider or physical therapist can give you tips on
getting a cane of proper length and how to walk with it.

One of the best ways to keep your muscles, bones, and joints
young is to stay active. This is also good for your diabetes. If you've
never been active, you can begin by exercising sitting down.

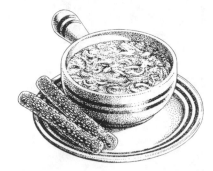

D *oes a meal plan have anything to do with my feet?*

▼

TIP:

Yes. You know that achieving near normal blood glucose levels can improve your chances of not having nerve damage or circulation problems. Part of managing your blood glucose is following a meal plan, along with daily exercise and diabetes medication if you need it. In addition, we know that what you eat affects your health including your skin, muscles, and bones. A meal plan that is unbalanced with too many processed foods (white flour, sugars, and fats) and too few vegetables and fruits leaves you with fewer weapons to use against bacteria and fungus on the skin. That is why healthy eating for people with diabetes is the same way everyone should eat. Especially important are the vitamins and the minerals that you can get from vegetables and fruits. You also want to be sure that you are getting enough calcium and magnesium for your bones. Ask for a referral to a registered dietitian (RD) if you need help designing or changing your meal plan to meet your needs and to get your blood glucose under control.

What you eat also affects your blood fats and plays an important part in circulation and peripheral vascular disease (see pages 98–104).

Chapter 2
SKIN CARE TIPS

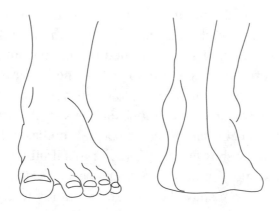

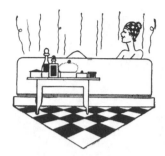

*W**hat is the best way for me to wash my feet?*

▼
TIP:

The best way to wash your feet is in the bathtub or shower. Wash your feet just like you wash the rest of your body. Make sure the water temperature is not too hot. Check the temperature with your elbow, not with your toes! You can use any good soap. If you have dry skin, you might want to try soap with moisturizer to combat dryness. Soap that is not milled is more moisturizing. (Milling removes glycerin to make the soap harder and easier to shape.)

If you prefer, or if you have to, you can wash your feet in a pan of water. Take the same precautions and be sure that the water is not too hot. It is not necessary to buy a special footbath. If you cannot use the bathtub or shower, any plastic or metal tub the size of a dishpan will work. You may have seen special footbaths in advertisements. Some have heating and vibrating features. If you have one, and you want to use it, you certainly can, but there are no special benefits to be gained.

Be sure to rinse your feet well and be sure to dry very well, especially between the toes. Use a soft fluffy towel to gently pat your feet dry.

Should I soak my feet?

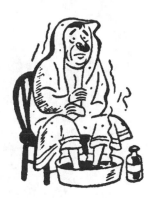

▼
TIP:

It is not necessary to soak your feet. In fact, prolonged soaking opens small cracks in your skin where germs can get in. That's how infections get started. Soaking also removes your natural skin oils. Repeatedly wetting and drying your feet can worsen dry skin problems, especially if you don't use a moisturizing lotion afterwards. For these reasons, soaking is not recommended.

If soaking your feet feels good, and you don't have any wounds on your feet, and the water is not too hot, and you don't stay in the footbath too long, and you use a moisturizing lotion afterwards, and you don't have any dry skin problems, you can probably get away with soaking your feet. However, from a health point of view, the risks of soaking your feet outweigh the benefits.

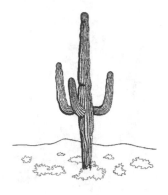

*W*hy do I have such dry skin on my feet?

▼
TIP:

As we age, skin may become thinner and dryer, so your dry skin may be from normal aging. People tend to have more dry skin in winter because of heating systems blowing dry air. Bathing with very hot water can also contribute to dry skin because it washes away natural skin oils. Harsh soaps and detergents also remove these oils.

People with diabetes can get a type of nerve damage called autonomic neuropathy. The autonomic nerves control blood flow, sweating, and skin moisture. People who have autonomic neuropathy may notice that their feet sweat less or not at all. This can cause severe dry skin.

Several other problems can cause dry skin of the feet. If your dry skin problem is not helped by regularly using a hand or body lotion, seek the advice of your health care provider.

Do I need to use skin lotions? What kind should I use and how often?

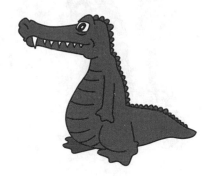

▼
TIP:

Yes, you need to moisturize dry skin to prevent itching and cracking, which keeps germs out. Moisturizers are packaged as creams, lotions, ointments, and oils. Any good body or hand lotion will do, as long as you remember to use it. Select the kind that you like and will actually use every day.

Avoid lotions with alcohol because it evaporates and takes moisture from the skin, which has a drying effect. Some people are sensitive to chemicals in highly perfumed or colored lotions, but there are lotions with no smell or color. Avoid lotions with lanolin if you are allergic to wool. Lotion with mineral oil as one of the main ingredients may not work as well as lotions containing olive oil, almond oil, jojoba oil, or vegetable oils. Aloe vera gel is another good moisturizer.

Ask your health care provider or pharmacist to recommend a moisturizer. You can get a prescription lotion if you have special problems or severe dry skin.

The best time to apply lotion is after a bath or a shower because it seals in the moisture your body has absorbed. Do not apply moisturizers between your toes. Apply lotion once a day, or if you have severe dry skin, two or three times a day. Keeping lotion in your sock drawer may help you remember to use it. You may prefer to apply lotion before going to bed. You can put on a pair of socks to keep the lotion off the sheets and help it soak in overnight.

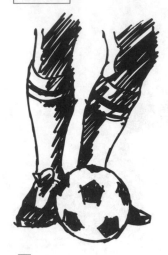

*How can I tell whether I have athlete's
foot fungus?*

▼
TIP:

The only way to tell for sure whether you have athlete's foot
fungus is for your health care provider to take a small skin
scraping and look at it under a microscope. However, when you
have itchy, burning, red, soggy, flaky, cracking, or dry scales
between your toes, it is most likely athlete's foot fungus. Therefore,
many providers will treat these symptoms as athlete's foot fungus
without actually testing for it.

Athlete's foot can also occur on the soles or sides of the feet with
many of the same symptoms and problems.

*W*hat should I do if I have athlete's
foot fungus?

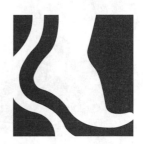

▼
TIP:

You can buy over-the-counter antifungal powders, sprays, and
creams. Do not use harsh chemicals like chlorine bleach. Bleach
does not kill the fungus and can burn your skin. Apply only a thin
layer of medicine. When athlete's foot flares up, apply the medication at least twice a day (morning and night) for at least 4 weeks.

See your provider if you have redness, swelling, or a warm area
anywhere on your foot, or if you see any pus. If you have fever or
chills or your blood sugar is higher than usual, you may have an
infection that needs to be treated.

Your provider can prescribe stronger antifungal creams and pills
for severe cases of athlete's foot. Unfortunately, it tends to come
back when treatment stops.

Remember to dry well between your toes. You can put on
antifungal foot powder. Some people find that lacing a little lamb's
wool between the toes helps keep that area dry. Don't use cotton
balls or tissues because they pack down and increase pressure
between the toes.

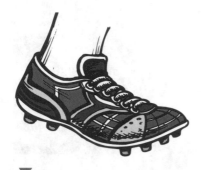

How can I prevent athlete's foot fungus?

▼
TIP:

There are several things you can do to prevent athlete's foot fungus from becoming a problem. The main one is to keep your feet clean and dry. Wear socks made of fibers that wick the moisture away from your skin. Put on a clean pair every day. If your feet get wet during the day, change socks more often.

Wear shoes with uppers made of leather or fabric that allow air to pass through. Allow your shoes to dry between wearings. If you have two pairs, alternate between them.

Almost all adults have athlete's foot fungus. There are lots of "normal" germs that just live on your skin, and athlete's foot fungus is one of these. It thrives in dark, warm, moist environments. It is mildly contagious and is passed on by contact in public showers and swimming areas, by sharing towels, or by using soiled bath mats. Wearing sandals at the local shower or pool has not been proven to prevent athlete's foot, but you should wear them to protect your feet from injury.

*W*hat should I do about foot odor?

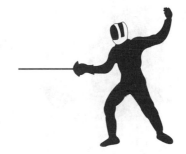

▼
TIP:

Foot odor is caused by the breakdown of bacteria on the skin. Daily bathing, changing socks, and keeping the feet clean and dry can control this. Using an antibacterial soap and a soft brush to gently scrub away dead skin may help. If your feet get wet during the day, you will need to change socks more often.

Always wear socks when you wear shoes. Wear shoes that allow air to circulate, not plastic or synthetic shoes. Dry out your shoes between wearings. Some foot odor problems are more smelly shoes than smelly feet. You may need to get new shoes.

If the problem continues, you might try an antiperspirant for feet or a foot powder designed to control foot odor. Special insoles with activated charcoal and socks that are designed to help control foot odor are available in large drugstores or from a foot care specialist.

Foot odor is sometimes a symptom of a serious problem such as a foot infection or foot ulcer that has gone undetected because of nerve damage. Inspect your feet carefully and if you detect a foot wound, see your provider immediately.

Why do my feet swell?

▼
TIP:

If both feet are swollen, it usually does not have much to do with your feet. If you have too much fluid in your system, it collects at the lowest part of the body due to gravity, and your feet and ankles swell. People with high blood pressure frequently have this kind of swelling. If your heart is too weak to pump blood around the body, the liquid parts of the blood tend to leak out of the blood vessels and collect in the lowest parts of the body. People with congestive heart failure have this kind of swelling. If your kidneys do not function well and you lose protein in your urine, your feet will swell.

Another cause of foot swelling is inactivity. When you are normally active during the day, the muscles in your legs help move blood and fluids back to the heart so they can recirculate. If you are sitting in a car or riding on an airplane all day, your leg muscles will not be working as much and fluid will pool in your feet and legs. That's why it's a good idea to get up and walk around every hour or two on an airplane or stop and walk around at a rest stop when you are in a car for long periods.

*W*hat should I do about foot swelling?

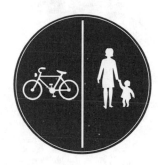

▼
TIP:

Elevate your feet and legs. Put your feet on a footstool, box, or another chair, or sit in a recliner with the footrest up. You can lie down on the couch and put your feet up on a pillow. Try to get your feet above the level of your heart. Any elevation is better than letting your feet hang down.

Another thing you can do is to stay active. Remember, when you are walking, the force of your contracting leg muscles helps blood and fluids return to the heart and keeps them from pooling in your feet and legs.

In some cases, you may be asked to take diuretics, often called "water pills." Water pills make you urinate a lot and leave less fluid in the system. That is how they lower blood pressure and make less work for a weak heart to do. Take your water pills as directed. Most people find it is best to take these pills first thing in the morning because they send you to the bathroom frequently. If you take them too close to bedtime, they might interrupt your sleep.

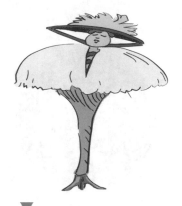

Should I wear support hose to control ankle swelling?

TIP:

Ask your health care provider because support hose should not be worn by people with poor circulation, skin disorders, infections, open wounds, or massive swelling. You must put them on before your feet or ankles swell, usually in the morning before you walk around much. Do not wear them to bed. Fluid will not accumulate in your feet while you are lying in bed.

Support hose come in several styles and colors for men and women and look like regular socks or stockings. Before buying below-the-knee support hose, measure around your calf at the widest part and from the floor to your knee. Do not guess. If you get the wrong size, they will be uncomfortable, and you will not wear them.

Your provider can advise you on how much "squeeze" you need. Hose come in different levels of compression—mild, moderate, and high. Some have high compression in the ankle and low compression in the calf. If they are too loose, they will not help, and if they are too tight, they cut off circulation. They can be custom knit to fit unusual leg shapes and fitted with zippers if you have trouble getting them on.

Chapter 3
NAIL CARE TIPS

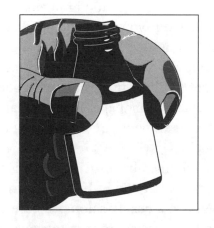

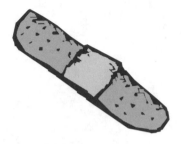

*C*an I cut my own toenails?

▼
TIP:

That depends on whether you can do it safely. Many people have trouble cutting their own toenails safely, especially if they are overweight or have arthritis or vision problems. If you can see and reach your feet well, and if you have good nail clippers, and you are careful, you can trim your own toenails. You could use a large nail file or emery board to file your nails. Filing is less risky than cutting. Nail files for artificial fingernails are good for toenail filing because they have coarser sandpaper than ordinary emery boards. If you have nerve damage or poor circulation or you can't see or reach your feet, ask for help.

If you have a family member or friend who is willing to help you, this might be the way to do it. If no podiatrist is available, another choice might be a beauty salon pedicure. Ask whether your provider has a nurse or assistant to trim toenails. In some communities, foot care is available through senior center programs. Almost all podiatrists will trim toenails. Medicare or health insurance may pay all or part of the cost for a podiatrist to trim your toenails if you have diabetes and meet certain criteria, such as having nerve damage and poor circulation.

*W*hat is the proper way to trim toenails when you have diabetes?

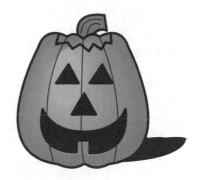

▼
TIP:

You may have seen instructions that say to cut your toenails straight across. However, this often leaves a sharp corner on the nail. It makes more sense to trim your nails with the contour of the toe, being sure all sharp edges are cut or filed smooth. The length of the toenail should be even with the end of the toe.

It is not a good idea to cut into the edges of the toenail or to try to treat ingrown toenails yourself. This sort of "bathroom surgery" is very risky for people with diabetes. The main point of safe toenail trimming is that if you do injure yourself, seek medical attention for any injury that does not heal promptly. If you have nerve damage or poor circulation and you cut yourself, see your provider right away. Do not wait until you develop an infection.

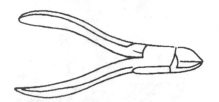

*W**hat is the best tool to use to trim my toenails?*

▼
TIP:

I prefer the nail clippers that look like a pair of wire cutters or pliers. They are available in large drugstores, beauty supply houses, and cutlery stores. It is not necessary to have a sterile tool, but your toenail nippers should be kept clean, dry, and sharp. When you use a tool that is dull, you have to put more pressure on the clippers, and you can injure yourself if they slip.

Do not use pocketknives, kitchen knives, sewing scissors, or your teeth, or pick at your toenails with your fingers. Once you have diabetes, it is too risky to try to cut your toenails with anything except a good pair of toenail clippers.

*W*hat should I do if I nick myself
while trimming my toenails?

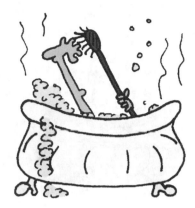

▼
TIP:

If you have nerve damage and poor circulation, go see your health care provider. If you don't, wash the injury with soap and water and pat it dry. It is not necessary to apply antiseptic creams to the wound. You may apply a bandage to keep it clean, but do not wrap the bandage tightly. Make it loose enough so that the circulation is not cut off if the toe or foot swells.

Do not be reassured if the wound does not hurt, because nerve damage may prevent you from feeling it. A wound that does not hurt may still be a serious injury.

Change the bandage and inspect the wound every day. Ask for help if you are having trouble seeing or caring for the injury. If you notice any redness, swelling, pus, or an area of increased warmth on your foot, or if the foot does not heal in a reasonable amount of time, report it to your health care provider right away. If you have an infection, you will need an antibiotic to cure it. The antibiotic creams that are currently available over the counter are not strong enough to cure an infection in a diabetic foot.

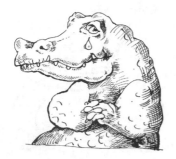

*W**hat should I do if I have very thick toenails?*

▼
TIP:

A very thick toenail can put lots of pressure on the toe and cause an ulcer, so it is a good idea to have it trimmed down or removed. Whether or not you can trim them yourself depends on how thick they are. Most people need help. It is best to go to a podiatrist or health care provider who is trained to trim thick nails and has special tools to do the job.

A fungus usually causes thick toenails. Creams, oils, and liquid drops are sold over-the-counter to treat fungal toenails. While these products may help soften the nail and retard the fungus somewhat, they usually do not make it go away.

There are prescription pills that may eliminate the fungus on your toenails; however, these medicines may affect your liver. You will need to have a blood test before you start the medicine and about 6 weeks into the 3-month treatment to check on your liver. If it is being damaged, you will have to stop taking the pills. If you want to cure fungal toenails, talk with your provider about these pills. Be aware that the fungus might return after you stop taking the medication.

Some patients report that keeping their glucose levels nearer normal helps with the toenail fungus problem.

*W*hat should I do if I have very curved
toenails?

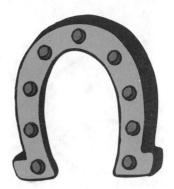

▼
TIP:

If you have deeply curved or ingrown nails, you may need help
trimming them. Do not try to cut or dig out the curving toenail.
You can injure yourself doing this. In addition, without the right
tools it is easy to leave a fragment of the nail that will turn into an
ingrown toenail and make the problem worse.

This kind of nail can be challenging even for professionals to cut.
It is best to go to a podiatrist or health care provider who is trained
to trim them. They have special tools that make it easier to trim very
curved toenails.

*W*hat should I do if I have ingrown toenails?

▼
TIP:

Ingrown toenails are a common problem for people with and without diabetes. This painful condition results when the nail grows into the skin. You're more likely to get it if you trim the toenails too short and cut down the sides of the toenail. Trim your toenails a bit longer, following the curve of the toe without leaving any sharp corners. If the toenail grows into the skin, it breaks the skin, and infection may develop. If the nail has simply been cut incorrectly, a podiatrist or other health care provider can remove the ingrown portion. He may give you an anesthetic to numb the pain. If you have nerve damage, the ingrown toenail may not hurt, but it certainly needs professional care.

If the problem keeps coming back, the podiatrist will numb the toe and remove a corner of the nail. Sometimes a chemical is put into the corner to keep the ingrown portion from coming back. Sometimes the whole toenail will have to be removed, and then a more normal toenail will usually grow back.

Chapter 4
SHOES AND SOCKS TIPS

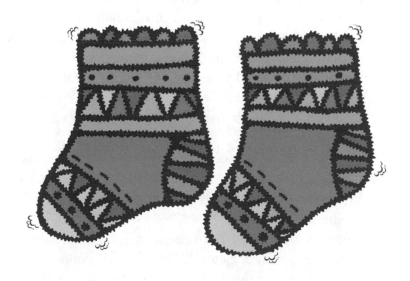

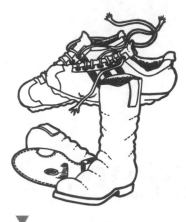

What are the best shoes to wear when you have diabetes?

▼
TIP:

Good quality athletic shoes or walking shoes are excellent choices. A lace-up shoe with a high rounded toe box is ideal. The upper part of the shoe should be a soft, breathable material such as leather or fabric instead of plastic or synthetic materials. Avoid sandals, clogs, thongs, or flip-flops, because they do not provide the same protection that a closed shoe does. If you have callus or a deformity, you need a shoe that redistributes the pressure on the sole of your foot. With a bunion or hammertoe, you may need extra-wide or extra-depth shoes.

If you have trouble tying laces, try shoes with Velcro™ fasteners. Most tie shoes can be converted to Velcro™ fasteners at a shoe repair shop. Elastic shoelaces allow you to get your shoes off and on without untying the laces.

Avoid tight, pointed shoes. High heels are not good for any foot—especially one with diabetes. They force the entire weight of the body onto the front of the foot, changing the shape, greatly increasing pressure, and causing ulcers. Look for a shoe that is shaped like a foot. While this sounds reasonable, it can be a challenging task, especially for women. It's worth the effort.

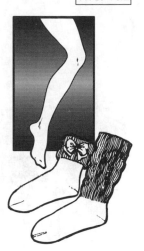

I have wall-to-wall carpeting; can I walk around bare foot or in my stocking feet?

▼
TIP:

No! Carpeting does not prevent you from stepping on pins, tacks, toys, dog bones, and whatever the cat brought in. Get a good pair of house shoes or slippers to protect your feet. The only time to go without shoes is when you are in bed or bathing. Even in the summer at a beach or pool, viruses, bacteria, and foreign bodies are lurking, just waiting for your bare feet. Always wear protective footgear.

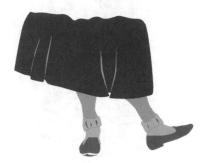

How can I tell whether my shoes fit?

▼
TIP:

One way is to purchase them from a trained shoe fitter (pedorthist). Have **both** feet measured every time you buy shoes, and shop for shoes in the afternoon or evening when your feet may be swollen. Your shoes need to fit all day. When you try on shoes, check that the ball of the foot rests in the widest part of the shoe. Walk a few steps, looking for signs of a poor fit, like the foot rolling over the sole, too much space between the heel and the back of the shoe, and notice that the shoe bends where your foot does. Be sure there is plenty of room for your toes. There should be a half-inch space between the longest toe and the end of the toe box, but the shoes should not slip. (The longest toe is not always the big toe.) Be sure the toe box is high enough and does not press on your toes.

Trace your foot, cut out the tracing, and place it on the sole of the shoe. Or put the sole of the shoe against the bottom of your foot. These can help you see whether the shape of the shoe matches the shape of your foot. If you have foot deformities or have had an ulcer that is now healed, you should have shoes prescribed and fitted or custom made by a podiatrist, orthopedic surgeon, or pedorthist. If you have nerve damage, your properly fitted new shoes may feel too big. Also remember that people's feet tend to get longer, wider, and flatter as years go by. You will not always wear the same size.

*M*y feet are different sizes; do I have
to buy two pairs of shoes?

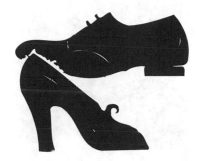

▼
TIP:

It is very common for one foot to be slightly larger or wider than
the other. If you need two different-sized shoes or if you have
only one foot, you might want to contact NOSE (the National Odd
Shoe Exchange) (see Resources). NOSE helps its members with
mismatched or odd-sized feet to find shoes. Some members are
matched with another member who has exactly the opposite shoe
size problem so that they can share shoe purchases rather than
having to buy two different-sized pairs to come up with one wearable
pair. Although it is rare, some stores will sell mismatched pairs.

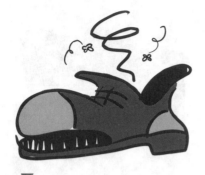

*W*hy should I inspect my shoes every day, and what am I looking for?

TIP:

Y̶ou are looking for anything that might injure your foot, especially if you have lost feeling in your feet. Look over the top and sole of the shoe, shake it out, and run your hand into it. Look and feel for any pebbles or foreign objects, or nails or tacks that may be coming through the sole. Look for cracked uppers or rough seams that could rub a blister. Replace shoes with worn or loose linings. If heels or soles are worn down, get new shoes or have them resoled so your foot is getting the support it needs.

*W*hat should I do if I need to wear special shoes for a special occasion?

▼
TIP:

The same principles that apply to fitting your everyday shoes apply to fitting special occasion shoes (see page 42). If you need to wear golf shoes, rented bowling shoes, ice skates, steel-toed work boots, ski boots, hiking boots, riding boots, or dress shoes to match your tuxedo or dress, you'll need to make sure they fit as well as possible. People prone to diabetes-related foot problems should not wear a strange pair of shoes for more than an hour or two. After the first hour, take a break, sit down, and check your feet for redness or pressure areas. Bring comfortable shoes to change into so you can avoid developing a blister.

If you need to wear high heels, wear the lowest heel possible (and no higher than 2 inches) for the shortest time possible. As soon as you get home or into your car, change into footwear that is more comfortable.

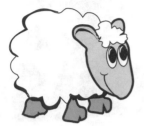

What are the best socks to wear?

▼
TIP:

Socks or stockings should be of breathable fibers such as cotton or wool, but they should also have acrylic or synthetic material that wicks moisture away from your skin. They should not be too tight or too loose and should fit without folds or wrinkles. Choose socks without seams. Garters or socks that bind may cut off circulation to your feet and legs. If the elastic at the top of your socks is too tight, cut a notch into the cuff of the sock.

Socks shaped like feet are preferable to tube socks, which tend to thin out over the heel and bunch up in the front. Change into clean socks daily. Throw away socks with holes. Repaired socks may have rough patches that can irritate your foot.

You can find extra large socks in big and tall shops, athletic stores, and department stores. Sports stores may have socks that are double knit on the bottom to provide an extra layer of cushioning. Just be sure that they don't make your shoes too tight.

Wear nylon stockings or panty hose for the shortest time possible. Nylon is not a breathable fabric (that's why they make raincoats out of it!). So change into some socks as soon as you can.

*D*o *I need custom shoes?*

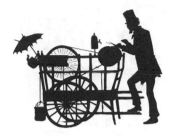

▼
TIP:

Most people with diabetes do not need custom-made shoes. However, if you are at risk for amputation, you may need a special shoe— for example, one with extra depth or special inserts. You are considered to be at risk for an amputation if you have already had a toe or partial-foot amputation, if you have a foot deformity, if you have had an ulcer that is now healed, or if you have diabetes-related foot problems. A podiatrist or other health care provider who can examine your feet would be the best person to advise you about this. A referral to a podiatrist may be necessary.

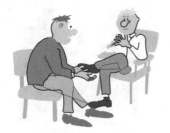

*W*ill Medicare pay for my therapeutic shoes?

▼
TIP:

Medicare pays for therapeutic footwear when you meet certain criteria and fill out the proper forms. This benefit covers custom-molded shoes, extra-depth shoes, inserts, and some shoe modifications. Your physician must certify that you are in a plan of diabetes care, have evidence of foot disease, and need therapeutic footwear. A podiatrist writes the prescription, and a podiatrist or pedorthist provides the shoes. You must buy the footwear from a qualified supplier and file the forms. You can get the forms from the prescription shoe stores, Medicare, or a podiatrist, or your provider may help you get them (*Medicare Carriers Manual*, section 2134 p2-85.1-2-86). Usually you have to pay for the shoes, and Medicare will reimburse up to 80% of the reasonable charge within limits. Ask about the charge and how much Medicare will pay when you order the shoes.

Although government programs can be time consuming, prescription footwear can be an important part of preventing foot problems.

*D*o I need insoles?

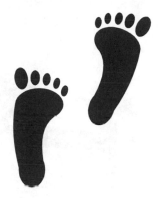

▼
TIP:

Maybe. You can relieve pressure on the soles of your feet by wearing a cushioning layer between your foot and the floor. If you wear thin-soled shoes or if you have high-pressure areas on your feet, it is a good idea to add insoles to your shoes. High-pressure areas are where calluses develop. Most ulcers begin under a callus. So if you can prevent or reduce the size of a callus, you may prevent getting an ulcer in that area, too.

These types of insoles are available in drugstores, grocery stores, sporting goods stores, and running shoe stores for less than $10 a pair. Running shoe stores also have insoles with extra arch support for $15 to $30. Be sure to check with your foot care specialist before buying these. An insole will raise your foot in the shoe, so be sure that you have plenty of room in the toe of the shoes. If your shoes are too tight with the insoles, you would do better with half-insoles that do not go under the toes. You'll need to change your insoles every 3–6 months to prevent foot odor and athlete's foot, and because the cushioning effect wears out.

If you have foot deformities or large calluses on your feet, you may need to have specially made inserts called orthotics to fit your feet (see page 51).

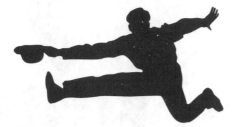

*D*o magnetic insoles offer any special benefits for people with diabetes?

▼
TIP:

We don't know yet. Although some people will swear that magnets relieve pain, improve circulation, reduce swelling, or provide other health benefits, at this time there are not enough scientific studies to back up these claims. Ordinarily when this is the case and the therapy is not harmful or expensive, health care providers will tell patients to try it and see what they think. However, some magnetic insoles have an uneven surface so they could possibly cause a sore or a foot ulcer in some people with diabetes who have high-pressure areas in their feet. People with diabetic nerve damage might not feel any discomfort from walking on these uneven surfaces and injure their feet. This means that the risks of magnetic insoles appear to outweigh the known benefits, so they are not recommended for people with diabetes to wear at this time. If you are really curious about them, you could try wearing them when you are not walking around, say for about 45 minutes when you are watching television or reading in bed.

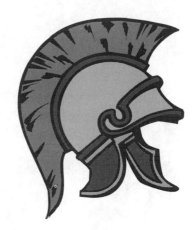

*W*hat are orthotics?

▼
TIP:

Orthotics are specially designed insoles that are worn inside your shoes to control the way your foot moves or to support painful areas of the foot. Often mistakenly called arch supports, they can do much more than that. Additions, top covers, extensions, or wedges can be added to the orthotics to hold your feet in a more stable position inside the shoe. This can help you walk normally, relieve foot pain, avoid calluses and corns, and even help with knee, hip, and lower back pain.

Orthotics are usually custom-made using a plaster model of your foot. They are made of a rigid material, like plastic, but some are made of leather or other soft materials. Graphite orthotics are durable and can be made very thin for comfort. Properly made orthotics are usually comfortable, but some people cannot stand to wear them. Work with your provider to get a pair that you will wear.

Orthotics can be expensive, so check to see whether your health plan will help you pay for them—often they will be covered. One pair may not fit inside all of your shoes, so you may want separate orthotics for dress shoes or sports. Orthotics must be replaced periodically, so ask the person who made them when you'll need new ones.

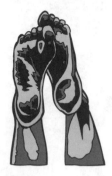

*D*o I need to wear orthotics?

▼
TIP:

You need orthotics if you have foot pain, a thick callus, or a change in foot shape that prevents you from walking normally. Sometimes people will have knee, hip, or lower back pain because of poor biomechanics in their feet and legs, and they need orthotics, too. If you cannot feel foot pain or whether your foot is in the correct position as you walk, you should have your gait evaluated by a professional. Orthotics are designed to fit the unique shape of your feet and to stabilize them in your shoes so your feet can work normally. If you have a foot deformity and poor sensation or circulation, orthotics can help keep your feet healthy. Discuss your options with a specialist such as an orthopedic foot surgeon or podiatrist. To get medically corrective foot orthotics you must have a prescription from a health care professional.

*W*hat is a pedorthist and do I need to
see one?

▼
TIP:

A pedorthist is a professional shoe fitter who has been trained in both foot anatomy and shoe construction. Pedorthists fill prescriptions for footwear and orthotics. A custom shoe store may have a pedorthist on staff. A nationally certified pedorthist may use the initials "C Ped" after his or her name.

If you have a severe foot deformity, you are probably already familiar with people trained in this specialty. If you have trouble getting shoes that fit properly or you need special adjustments to your shoes because your feet are changing shape or you're losing feeling in your feet, it might be a good idea to see a pedorthist.

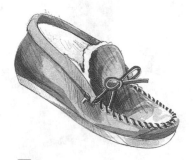

I have had a partial foot amputation. Can I just put padding in my shoes and continue to wear the shoes I wore before the surgery?

▼
TIP:

Maybe. You need to have your foot examined by a podiatrist or an orthopedic surgeon to see where the pressure points are and whether there are any new ones since the surgery. An amputation "creates" a foot deformity, and it is important to fit your shoes properly so that they do not rub a blister or cause a buildup of callus. You may need orthotics or a specially made shoe.

Chapter 5
TREATING
MINOR PROBLEMS

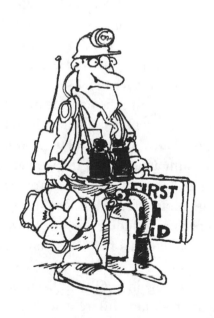

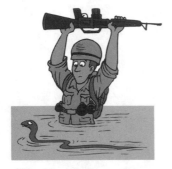

I *have a blister on my foot, what should*
I do?

▼
TIP:

If you have neuropathy or poor circulation, see your health care provider immediately! Don't wait until it gets infected. Then the first thing to do is to stop wearing the offending shoe. Wash the area with warm water and mild soap and dry well. Do not break the blister—this can allow germs to get under the skin. Cover the blister with a dry bandage. If the blister breaks, leave the loose skin as a covering over the wound until it heals. It is not necessary to apply antiseptics, antibiotic ointments, or chemicals to the blister.

Inspect the blistered area daily. If there is redness, tenderness, swelling, pus, or a warm area around the wound after the first day, you may be getting an infection. See your provider to get antibiotics. Over-the-counter antibiotic creams are not strong enough to treat a foot infection in a person with diabetes. If the wound is deep, gets larger, or does not heal within a few days, have it checked immediately.

Don't wear the shoes again until the blister is entirely healed. You might need extra padding, different socks, or something else to keep them from rubbing. Wear the shoes for a short while, then check your feet for signs of another blister. It is better to throw them away than to continue wearing shoes that injure your feet.

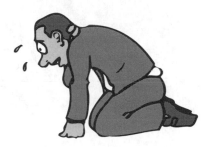

I wore well-fitting shoes and cushioned socks, and I still got a blister. How is this possible?

▼
TIP:

A blister is usually a sign of friction. If your shoes do not rub and you are getting blisters on your feet for no apparent reason, check with your health care provider. There is a rare diabetic complication called diabetic bullae. Bulla (bullae is the plural) is the medical term for a fluid-filled blister. The layers of the skin just separate and fill with clear fluid for no apparent reason, usually on the hands and feet. There can be several small blisters, just one, or sometimes a very large blister. There is no special treatment for diabetic bullae, just care for it as you would any other blister.

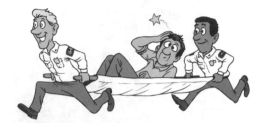

I *stubbed my toe, what should I do?*

▼

TIP:

Well, that depends on how much you have injured it. While a stubbed toe can be excruciatingly painful, the actual injury can vary from minor to severe. If you don't have peripheral vascular disease, put ice on the injury and elevate it higher than your heart to relieve the swelling and pain. Is the toe in an abnormal position or do you have continued pain, swelling, or an inability to put weight on the foot? Then you need to see your health care provider for an X ray of your foot to make sure that you have not broken any bones. If you neglect a fracture, particularly of the big toe, this can result in a painful deformity. You need early treatment to prevent this from occurring. Sometimes people with nerve damage do not feel pain and can injure a foot or toe quite severely without knowing it. If you have nerve damage, check your feet carefully with your eyes and your hands after any injury to see how bad it is.

If blood accumulates under the toenail, it can put pressure on the toe. You may need to visit your health care provider to have the pressure relieved. Do not try to relieve it yourself by puncturing the nail or performing any other home surgery. When you have diabetes, it is best to have a health care provider treat all foot injuries.

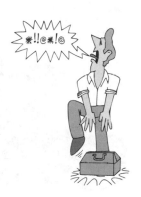

I stepped on a nail, what should I do?

▼

TIP:

If you have neuropathy and poor circulation, see your health care provider right away. Puncture wounds are a serious matter, especially when you have diabetes. Nails and other sharp objects do not have to be rusty to cause lockjaw (tetanus) or to cause an infection in your foot. Punctures through shoes are especially dangerous because sometimes a little rubber from the sole of the shoe is carried into the wound and causes an especially nasty type of infection.

Wash the area with warm water and mild soap and dry well. Cover the wound with a dry bandage. It is not necessary to apply antiseptics or antibiotic ointments. Change the bandage daily. If the bandage sticks when you attempt to remove it, apply a little warm water first. Inspect the wound every day and if you see any redness, swelling, pus, or drainage, or you have unexplained high blood sugar, report it to a health care provider immediately.

All adults should have tetanus booster shots repeated at least every 10 years. If you are not sure when you had your last tetanus booster, it is safe to have another one when you are injured.

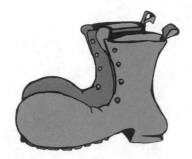

My toenail fell off, what should I do?

▼
TIP:

After a toenail injury, it is very common for the nail to fall off. Sometimes this happens with very thick fungal nails. It will usually grow back within 12–18 months. Keep the area clean and dry while waiting for the new nail to grow back. Protect it from any further damage by not going barefoot and by wearing shoes that have plenty of room for your toes. The nail-growing cells may have been damaged during the injury, so sometimes the new toenail will be a different shape.

*W*hat does it mean if my toes curl over?

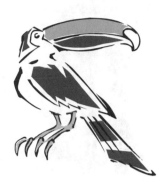

▼
TIP:

It means that you have had a change in the position of the foot bones and have tight tendons in the toe. Toes that are curled or bent are called hammertoes, claw toes, or mallet toes. You may have one or several. A foot deformity like this can set you up for calluses and possibly an ulcer because hard tissue, called a corn, will grow on top of or on the tip of the curving toe. The corn is nature's way of protecting the joint from irritation when it rubs against your shoe. Sometimes toe deformities are very painful. To deal with a toe deformity, you can change shoes, pad the toe, trim the corn, wear orthotics, or have surgery on the foot. If you use corn pads, be sure to buy ones that do not contain any chemicals.

Inspect your feet every day and see your health care provider or podiatrist whenever the corn needs trimming or becomes irritated. Inspect both the top of the toe where the corn develops and the tip of the toe, which can also rub and develop a callus.

Try switching to shoes that have a soft, rounded toe box and a soft insole under the toes to decrease irritation to the toe. Surgery can release the tendons and relax the toe or put the bones in a correct position. But you may also need orthotics to address any biomechanical problem.

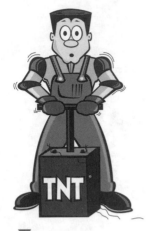

*C*an I use over-the-counter corn and
callus removers?

▼
TIP:

N o, you really should not use these products when you have
diabetes. Usually the manufacturer will say "not for use by
people with diabetes" on the product. Corn and callus removers,
corn plasters, and similar products are harsh chemicals, usually acids.
They decrease the buildup of hard skin by softening and burning
away the corn or callus. If you have diabetic nerve damage, you
might not be able to feel it if the chemicals burned too much or got
on the surrounding normal skin. It is dangerous for a person with
diabetes to get any breaks in the skin because of the risks of
infection and difficulty with healing. Therefore, you should avoid
putting harsh chemicals on your feet.

You might try a green clay poultice to soften corns and calluses,
but you really should try to determine what is causing them. See
your regular provider or a podiatrist if you have a corn or callus that
needs to be treated.

*W*hat should I do about a corn
between my toes?

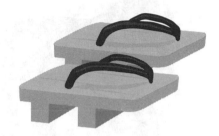

▼
TIP:

Corns between the toes that touch each other are called soft corns or kissing corns. Bones in adjacent toes rubbing together cause these corns. Shoes that squeeze the toes together aggravate soft corns. Sometimes they are very painful.

You can change shoes, add padding, and have surgery for soft corns. Switch to shoes that have a soft and high rounded toe box that does not press your toes together. You can buy special toe separator pads made of soft foam rubber or loosely lace some lamb's wool between the toes to decrease the rubbing. Do not use cotton or tissues between the toes because these materials can pack down and actually increase the pressure. Inspect your feet every day, including between the toes. See your podiatrist or another health care provider if you think the soft corn needs to be trimmed, or if it is irritated or ulcerated.

Early surgery to correct the problem causing the corn is often the best solution to prevent the corn from occurring. Elective foot surgery is often more important for people with diabetes than for the general population. Many foot ulcers begin as a callus or corn.

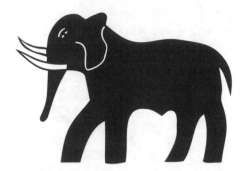

*W*hat should I do about a
callus on the bottom of
my foot?

▼
TIP:

Try to decrease the high pressure on that spot by wearing shoes
with a soft insole and a cushioned outer sole. Don't wear house
shoes with little cushioning or go barefoot because this will make
the callus worse. A hard callus is like having a rock in your shoe.
The tissue beneath the callus can become damaged, and most foot
ulcers occur there. You need to be evaluated by a professional to see
what is causing the callus.

To deal with a callus you can change shoes, get orthotics, moisturize
the skin, trim the callus, or have surgery. If it is very thick, you may
need orthotics. In any case, moisturizing the callused area with a
good lotion keeps it soft. A green clay poultice will also soften it.
Callus can be sanded down with an emery board, callus file, or a
pumice stone. It may be easier to remove after a bath or shower
when the skin is still damp. Go easy and do not injure yourself by
scrubbing too hard. Buff the area a little every other day rather than
try to remove the callus all at once. Never try to remove a callus by
cutting or trimming it with a razor blade. See your podiatrist or
health care provider for ongoing callus care.

*W*hat should I do about a wart on the bottom of my foot?

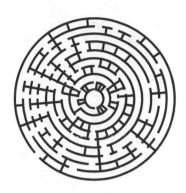

▼
TIP:

Plantar warts are caused by the papilloma virus, which gets under the skin on the bottom of the foot. In some people, plantar warts disappear without any treatment. In others, plantar warts hang around for years even when they are treated.

There are many home remedies for plantar warts, but the best solution is to see your health care provider or a podiatrist. Sometimes it is difficult even for professionals to tell the difference between a plantar wart and a callus. There are several treatments for plantar warts including leaving them alone if they are not painful. They can be trimmed, padded, or removed with chemicals, burned with liquid nitrogen, or removed by surgery. It is important not to leave a painful scar on the bottom of the foot that can affect walking, so it is best not to try any of these treatments by yourself.

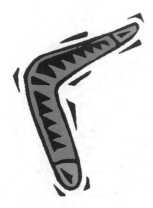

*W*hat is a bunion? What should I do if I have one?

▼
TIP:

A bunion is called hallux valgus. Hallux is the medical name for the big toe, and valgus is a word that means turning away from the midline of the body. A bunion is a deformity in the joint of the big toe causing the toe to point away from the arch instead of straight ahead. There is usually an unsightly bump on the inside of the foot. It is believed that uneven weight distribution during walking and stresses in the joints cause bunions and that they tend to run in families. Wearing shoes with pointed toes probably contributes to developing bunions.

If you have a painful bunion or it is difficult to get your shoes to fit, discuss what to do with your health care provider. Don't put it off. You may need special shoes, orthotics, or padding. Some bunions need surgical correction. If you have good circulation, get the surgery done. Early surgery is often the best treatment for people with diabetes. Modern bunion surgery not only removes the bump but also attempts to correct the mechanical problem that caused it so the bunion does not grow back. Bunion surgery can take about 6 weeks to heal, so you will want to have good blood glucose control before and after the surgery to encourage healing.

Chapter 6
EXERCISE TIPS

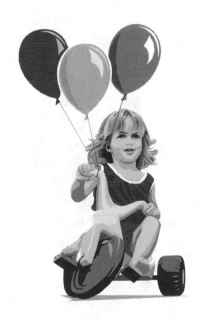

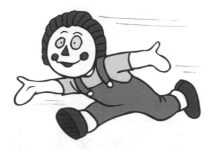

*W*hat foot precautions should I
follow when walking, running,
or jogging?

▼
TIP:

Have a foot exam to discover any deformity, lack of feeling, or poor circulation. Wear clean socks and good-quality walking or running shoes to prevent injury. Always take the time to warm up and do slow stretches to prepare your muscles and tendons—especially your Achilles' tendons. Cool down and stretch after the exercise activity and inspect your feet for redness, blisters, or callus buildup. If you have pain during exercise, stop and try to figure out what is wrong. You may need orthotics to help your feet work normally during physical activity—especially if you are active and have knee pain or pain in the arch or heel area of your foot (plantar fasciitis).

If you have a loss of feeling in your feet, limit repetitive weight-bearing exercises such as jogging and stair climbers because of the high pressure on your feet and possible injury that you wouldn't be able to feel. Be careful of hot sand and pavement around pools and sports courts. Even if you wear thin-soled sandals and water shoes, your feet may still get burned.

If you have a foot ulcer, do not do weight-bearing exercise so it can heal. When the ulcer has healed, try to discover what caused it and take special precautions when exercising to prevent it from coming back.

Drink plenty of water when you are exercising.

*W*hat forms of exercise are good for people with diabetic foot complications?

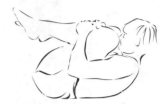

▼
TIP:

Short periods of walking can actually improve circulation in your legs and feet by forcing the blood vessels to work harder and expand. In fact, this is the recommended exercise for people with intermittent claudication. Walking is good for your heart and for your diabetes control too. Two 20-minute walks a day is ideal.

If you have lost much of the feeling in your feet, you can participate in non-weight-bearing exercises, such as swimming, bicycling, or rowing, and upper body exercises, such as weight lifting, and range of motion and stretching exercises. You can do yoga. You will achieve your best level of fitness if you do several different types of exercise during the week. For example, you can do aerobic exercise one day, stretching exercises the next, and strength-building exercises the next day. If you row or bicycle on a machine, take care that the foot straps don't injure your feet. In a pool, you may want to wear aqua shoes to protect your feet.

Remember that your household chores, such as vacuuming and gardening, count as aerobic exercise, too.

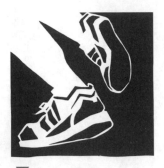

Should I wear special shoes when exercising?

▼
TIP:

Yes, you should always wear good-quality athletic shoes made for the activity you are doing. This means wearing running shoes for running, golfing shoes for golfing, and bowling shoes for bowling. Almost every sport is associated with a special type of shoe appropriate to the particular activity. These shoes are important for preventing injury. And they may help you perform better and enjoy the sport more! If you are in doubt about which shoes to wear, a good running shoe offers support and stability to protect your feet from injury.

Chapter 7
IDENTIFYING
MAJOR PROBLEMS

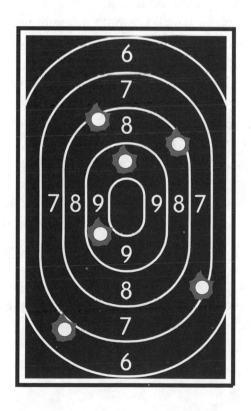

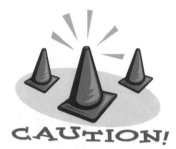

*H*ow do I know when I have a foot
ulcer?

CAUTION!

▼

TIP:

A foot ulcer is an open sore somewhere on your foot. The term "ulcer" refers to a wound or hole in the skin. We often hear about a stomach ulcer, which is a hole in the lining of the stomach. A foot ulcer is a break in the skin that is usually, but not always, shaped like a crater. Foot ulcers often occur in high-pressure areas, so it is common to find one under a callus or surrounded by callus. The most common foot ulcer locations are on the bottom or side of the big toe and on the ball of the foot, especially under the big toe joint. The ball of the foot under the little toe joint is also a common place for foot ulcers. However, diabetic foot ulcers can occur anywhere on the feet. Be aware that the actual break in the skin can be very small, but a larger ulcer may be hidden from view under the surrounding callus or skin. This is why it is important to have your foot inspected by a professional if you think you might have a foot ulcer.

The only way for you to know whether you have a foot ulcer is by seeing it or feeling it. That is why we ask people with diabetes to inspect their feet carefully every day.

*H*ow do I avoid getting foot ulcers?

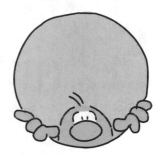

▼
TIP:

*Y*ou can take two very important steps to protect your feet. Control your blood sugar levels as well as you can. Inspect your feet every day and get regular medical attention at least several times a year. There is no magic to avoiding foot complications. The key is to develop a routine that includes some commonsense everyday attention to your feet.

- Keep your feet clean and dry.
- Wear well-fitting shoes and socks.
- Don't go barefoot.
- Don't soak your feet.
- Don't put lotion between your toes, but put it on the rest of your foot.
- Get monofilament testing at least once a year.
- Treat calluses aggressively by seeing a foot care specialist.
- Get any injury to your foot seen right away!

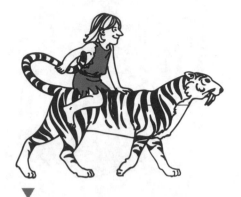

What should I do if I get a foot ulcer?

▼ TIP:

Have any foot ulcer examined by a health care professional, and once you have received treatment, the wound should begin to heal in a week or two. Keep the wound clean and dry and covered with a bandage. Inspect it daily. You must follow the treatment plan. Usually the treatment is to trim or cut away (debride) the dead tissue, to apply a dressing every day, and, if the wound is infected, to take antibiotics. It is likely that you will be asked to change your shoes. You must not walk on an infected foot. Use bed rest, crutches, or a wheelchair, but stay off that foot.

If the wound is not improving after a week or two, let your health care provider know. Be sure that you are doing all you can to follow the treatment plan and help your foot to heal.

*T*his foot ulcer is not getting better, what
should I do?

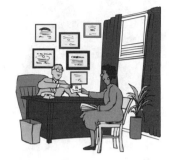

▼
TIP:

If you are following the care plan, taking antibiotics, and not
walking on the ulcer but it still isn't healing, ask your health care
provider for a referral to a foot care specialist. You may also need to
be evaluated by a vascular surgeon to see whether surgery might
restore circulation to the foot and help heal the ulcer. As a person
with diabetes, you must be in charge of your own health care. Ask
for a second opinion or to be referred to a specialist if your wound
is not healing. Nonhealing ulcers lead to amputation, so get the help
you need.

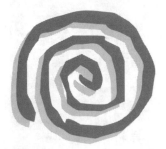

*H*ow do I know whether I have an *infection?*

▼
TIP:

Some signs of infection are

- redness
- swelling
- increased warmth
- pain, tenderness, or limited motion of the affected part
- pus or drainage from the wound

If you have one or two of these signs, have a health care provider check your wound to determine whether you have an infection.

Other signs that an infection has spread beyond the wound are fever, chills, or an unusually high blood sugar. If you have any of these signs, you need to be seen immediately and should go to an emergency room if your regular health care provider cannot see you right away.

Chapter 8
COMPLICATIONS—
NERVE DAMAGE

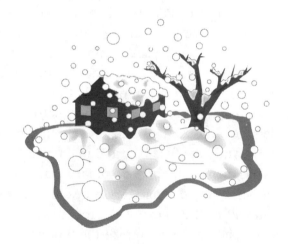

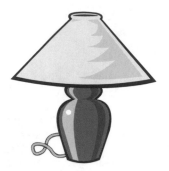

W^{hat is peripheral neuropathy?}

▼
TIP:

Peripheral neuropathy is the name for damage to motor and sensory nerves. Motor and sensory nerves help you move and touch the world around you. "Peripheral" means at the edges or away from the center. In this case, the feet are farthest from the center of the body. "Neuro" means nerves and "pathy" means "a disorder of." Because the longest nerves are usually affected first, symptoms such as tingling, burning, or numbness appear first in the feet and hands.

If you think of the nervous system as the electrical system in your house, then the wires to the lights and appliances would be the peripheral nerves, while the fuse box and main cable would be the central nervous system (the brain and spinal cord).

When motor nerves are damaged, muscles in your foot can become weak and allow the shape of the foot to change. Toes can curl up and the fat pad on the bottom of the foot can shift and no longer protect the skin on the bottom of the foot. Those bones can get very close to the skin and can cause calluses. The sensory nerve damage prevents you from feeling pain, so the callus can become an ulcer without you knowing it.

How does diabetes cause nerve damage?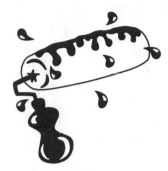

▼
TIP:

Nobody really knows. It is pretty certain that higher than normal blood sugar levels are part of the cause. We do know that keeping your blood sugar in control can lower your chances of getting neuropathy, that people with high blood sugar are more likely to have neuropathy, and that the longer a person has diabetes, the more likely he or she is to have neuropathy.

There are several theories about how blood sugar affects nerves. It is possible that sugar coats the proteins in the nerves and that the sugar-coated proteins no longer function normally. Or, it might be that high blood sugar levels interfere with chemical events in the nerves. Maybe high blood sugar levels damage the insulation layer of cells around the nerves. It might be that high blood sugar levels damage the tiny blood vessels that supply the nerves. Then the nerves would not get enough oxygen and nutrients, and this could cause problems.

Researchers are working to understand the causes of neuropathy and to find treatments to avoid the damage that it does.

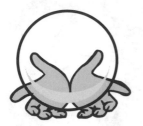

How do I know whether I have peripheral neuropathy?

▼
TIP:

If you have had diabetes for more than 10 years and you have not kept your blood sugar levels close to near normal levels, you likely have some symptoms of nerve damage. It affects as many as 75% of all people with diabetes. Do you have muscle weakness, cramps, and feelings in your feet and legs such as numbness, tingling, pins and needles, and burning sensations? Do your feet bother you more at night? Have you had any episodes of fainting or vomiting or had a change in bowel habits, bladder control, or sexual functioning? These systems can be affected by diabetic nerve damage too.

There is no one specific test for diabetic nerve damage. Generally if you have two or more symptoms and one of the simple tests for loss of sensation is positive (you cannot feel the touch of a plastic wire or a vibrating tuning fork on the bottom of your foot, see page 82), you will be considered as having neuropathy.

*D*oes diabetes cause more than one kind of neuropathy?

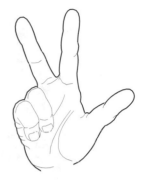

▼
TIP:

Yes, diabetic nerve damage can affect three kinds of nerves in your body: nerves you feel with (sensory neuropathy), nerves that go to the muscles (motor neuropathy), and nerves that control automatic body activities such as blood flow and digestion (autonomic neuropathy). With sensory nerve damage you may not be able to feel heat and cold and may have tingling, pain, or numbness. You may not be able to sense where your feet are and be more likely to fall. With motor nerve damage, muscles are weakened and you are more likely to develop foot deformities such as hammertoes.

Damage to autonomic nerves can affect major systems in your body, such as the heart, stomach, or sexual organs. It can affect heart rate and blood pressure. It can cause gastroparesis and erectile dysfunction. This type of nerve damage can also interfere with the functioning of your bladder, eyes, sweat glands, and hypoglycemia awareness (symptoms of low blood sugar).

The best way to try to prevent nerve damage is to keep your blood sugar levels closer to normal. Getting better blood sugar control can help relieve symptoms of ongoing neuropathy, but you may not be able to reverse extensive damage, such as you find in completely numb feet.

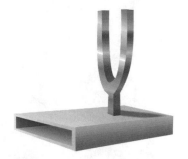

*W*hat kinds of tests do I need for
peripheral neuropathy?

▼
TIP:

Many people with neuropathy already know that their feet are
numb. Most people who have symptoms of neuropathy (pain,
numbness, tingling), especially if their symptoms are worse at night,
can be considered to have neuropathy. However, you could have
neuropathy from a cause other than diabetes, such as vitamin
deficiencies, thyroid disease, poisons (alcohol, lead, mercury, or
arsenic), and several other diseases. Your provider may want to be
sure that you do not have any of these other problems.

One of the most common tests is for the health care provider to
touch your feet with a plastic wire called a monofilament. If you
cannot feel the wire, you are considered to have nerve damage.
Similar tests check whether you can feel a pin prick, a wisp of
cotton stroked across the foot, or the vibration of a tuning fork.

If there is confusion about the nerve damage, some people might
need a nerve conduction study. On rare occasions, a nerve biopsy in
which a small piece of nerve tissue is examined under a microscope
is done. If you are asked to have tests for neuropathy, ask your
provider to explain the tests to you.

A re there any treatments for peripheral neuropathy?

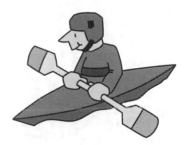

▼
TIP:

The best treatment is to get your blood sugar levels under control. Studies show that good blood sugar control can also help prevent the nerve damage that you already have from getting worse. Take note that if you should go on insulin or a sulfonylurea and improve your blood sugar control, the pain may increase for a little while, until your body becomes accustomed to the lower blood sugar levels.

Medications such as antidepressants, anticonvulsants (seizure medicine), muscle relaxants, local anesthetics (such as a lidocaine patch), anti-inflammatory drugs, vitamins, evening primrose oil, and capsaicin creams made from hot peppers have been used to treat neuropathy symptoms. Physical therapy treatments such as stretching exercises, massage, and electrical nerve stimulation have also been tried. Although studies of these therapies report some improvement in painful symptoms for some patients, there is no single treatment that works for everyone. It may be difficult to get complete relief. Discuss your symptoms with your provider and try the treatment you both think might work. If that treatment doesn't help, let your provider know so you can try another.

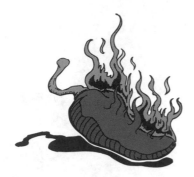

How can capsaicin cream help relieve my neuropathy pain?

▼
TIP:

Capsaicin is a substance found in hot peppers. Capsaicin cream removes a chemical from the nerve ends below your skin and may interrupt your feeling of pain. Apply it lightly several (3–5) times a day. Wash your hands carefully after applying capsaicin—you would not want to get hot pepper cream in your eyes! When you first use capsaicin, you may have a stinging or burning sensation that should disappear in a few days.

Buy only a small amount to try. Do not use capsaicin if you are sensitive or allergic to hot peppers. Capsaicin cannot be used on damaged or irritated skin, wounds, or rashes. Don't put tight clothing or bandages over the cream. Use it 3–4 times a day for 3–4 weeks before deciding whether it is working. Ask your provider or pharmacist if you have questions.

Purchase a product made by a reputable company. Some natural product companies and herbalists make up their own concoctions containing extracts of hot peppers, but the strength and purity of the drug is usually not consistent.

*M*y feet are getting more sensitive, not
less. How can this be nerve damage?

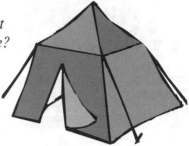

▼
TIP:

W hen the nerves are in the process of being damaged, many
strange signals can be sent up the nerve pathways, including
feeling as though your feet are more sensitive than they should be.
Some people find it painful for bedsheets to touch their feet. If you
experience this, placing a hoop or a box over the end of the bed so
that the sheet is kept off your feet might provide you some relief.

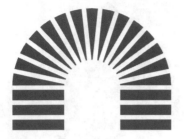

What can I do for the numbness in my feet?

▼
TIP:

This is a very serious condition. The main thing to do about numbness in your feet is to realize that you have it. Most people go to the doctor because their foot hurts. Yours never will. You **must** check your feet by touching them with your hands and by looking at them every day! Controlling your blood sugar as well as possible may help prevent the numbness from getting worse. Get your shoes fitted properly, if necessary by a pedorthist, and find out whether you need special shoes to protect your feet. Check your shoes before each wearing for foreign objects, nails, or anything that would injure your foot. Be sure your socks are not wrinkled or twisted. You may want to switch to socks without a toe seam because the seam can put too much pressure on your toes.

If you find the numbness is uncomfortable, discuss treatments for neuropathy with your health care provider. Whenever there is any injury to your feet or a change in shape or the skin, see your foot care specialist right away. Do **not** wait until an infection develops!

*W*hat does it mean if it feels like my feet are
*burning, tingling, or something is crawling
on my feet but nothing is there?*

▼
TIP:

Burning, tingling, or crawling sensations on the feet or legs may
be a sign that diabetic nerve damage is occurring. The first thing
to do is to check to make sure there is no obvious cause for this sensation. If you find this sensation uncomfortable, you may want to talk
with your health care provider about possible treatments for neuropathy.
You may also want to go over your diabetes care plan to see whether
it is helping you keep your blood sugar levels where you want them
to be.

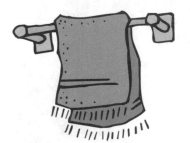

*M**y feet are sweating more, what can I do?*

My feet are sweating more, what can I do?

▼
TIP:

An increase in foot sweating can be a sign that diabetic nerve damage is occurring. If you have sweaty feet, wear shoes made of leather or fabric that "breathes." Avoid shoes made of plastic or synthetic materials. Try to change your shoes during the day. If that is not possible, rotate between two pairs of shoes, wearing one on even days and the other on odd days. (Keeping your feet dry helps you avoid fungal infections, but it is also important to avoid excessively dry skin that may crack.)

Wear socks that wick the moisture away from your skin (special acrylic blends). You can find two- and three-layer socks designed to absorb sweat in sports stores. Change socks frequently: at least daily and maybe two or three times a day if necessary. If you have to wear nylon stockings, change into socks as soon as you can. Can you wear cotton tights instead?

You may have to try an antiperspirant containing aluminum chloride, such as "Drysol" that is available with a prescription. An antiperspirant can dry and irritate your skin so use it sparingly and only as a last resort. Follow the directions on the package and stop using the product immediately if you experience any skin irritation.

*W*hy don't my feet sweat anymore?

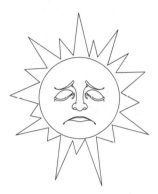

▼
TIP:

A decrease in foot sweating can also be a sign that diabetic nerve damage is occurring in the nerves that control sweating. They just don't work normally. However, foot sweating also tends to decrease as we age, especially if we become less active. Wearing different shoes or socks can affect foot sweating, too. You may have recently started wearing shoes that do not hold in moisture, so your feet are drier.

The problem with a decrease in foot sweating, whatever the cause, is that the foot skin tends to become very dry and prone to cracking. It is a good idea to use a moisturizing cream or lotion on your feet (but not between the toes) if you have dry skin.

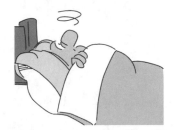

*W*hy do my feet bother me more at night?

▼

TIP:

Nobody really knows the answer to this question. It is thought that the symptoms of diabetic nerve damage (pain, burning, tingling, numbness, etc.) are just more noticeable at night because the nerves of the feet and legs are not getting the other signals that they get during the day when you are up and about and walking more. Also during the day, you get a broad spectrum of sensory signals from things you see, hear, taste, touch, and smell that keep you busy and distracted from the neuropathy symptoms.

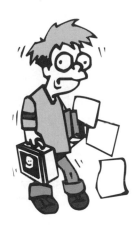

Can an unsteady gait be related to diabetic nerve damage?

▼
TIP:

Yes! When a person has loss of feeling in his or her feet, the positioning system of the body does not get normal responses about where the feet are being placed. This can cause the person to feel unsteady or to trip and stumble. People with nerve damage tend to walk slower with a wide-based gait compared to how they walked before having neuropathy. However, an unsteady gait can be a sign of other problems too, some of which can be quite serious. If you are having trouble with your balance or walking, talk with your provider.

If your trouble is due to nerve damage, it may be time to get a cane. Your provider or physical therapist can help you get the right length and give you tips on how to walk with a cane. A physical therapist can also teach you balance exercises and how to increase awareness of the position of your feet.

Sometimes diabetes-related muscle weakness can contribute to unsteadiness in walking. Your provider or physical therapist can show you muscle strengthening exercises. Some people need a lightweight brace or ankle support to stabilize the ankles when muscle weakness is the problem.

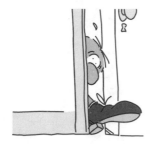

Why does diabetic nerve damage affect the feet first?

▼
TIP:

Nobody really knows the answer to this question. It is known that the longest nerves are affected first and the longest nerves are those traveling to the feet. A nerve has a cell body and then a long nerve fiber extending from the cell body. It looks a little like a root from a plant. Some people think that the long nerves are affected first because the small nerve fibers at the end of long nerves are the most distant from their cell bodies and are, therefore, the most easily damaged. Other people think that all the nerves are affected more or less equally and symptoms appear in the long nerves first because there are more of these nerves to be damaged.

Chapter 9
COMPLICATIONS—
POOR CIRCULATION

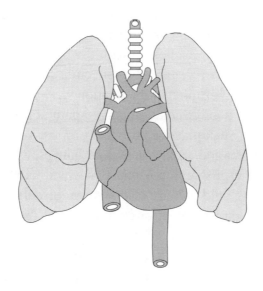

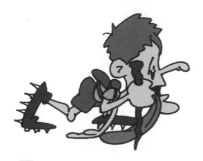

*H*ow do I know when I have poor circulation in my feet and legs?

▼
TIP:

The hallmark sign of poor circulation is pain or cramping in the calf or the thigh (usually the calf) that occurs when you walk a short distance. This pain is a sign that the muscles are not getting enough oxygen. If you slow or stop and rest for a few minutes, the oxygen supply usually catches up with the demand and then you can walk a little further before the pain reoccurs. The medical term for this condition is "intermittent claudication."

Other signs of poor circulation can be pain at rest, nonhealing ulcers, absent or weak pulses in the feet or legs, a decrease in blood pressure in the feet and legs, or a lack of hair growth on the lower legs. A blue or purplish color, especially when your feet are hanging down, and having cold feet are also signs of circulation problems.

If you think you have poor circulation to the feet, ask your provider to evaluate it. Poor circulation is caused by a blockage in the arteries supplying blood to the feet. The blockage may need to be removed or bypassed with vascular surgery. A simple treatment is to walk every day. This exercise can force the blood vessels to expand and improve the circulation in your feet and legs.

I *have varicose veins. Does that mean I*
have poor circulation?

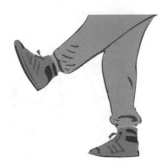

▼
TIP:

Varicose veins are a different type of poor circulation—a poor
return of blood to the heart. Your feet are supplied with blood
by arteries that carry blood down to them. Veins carry blood from
the feet back to the heart. When you stand up, gravity tends to pull
blood down towards your feet. Leg veins have valves in them to
prevent this from happening. However, if the valves are damaged or
too far apart, they do not close properly. This causes varicose veins,
which tend to get very full and widen with blood. Varicose veins
may look like blue snakes or rivers under the skin. Some of the fluid
in the blood leaks out through very small veins (capillaries) and
causes swelling. This pooling of blood can cause ulcers on the legs,
but these are different from diabetic foot ulcers. Anyone can have
varicose veins and leg ulcers.

Wearing support hose and exercise are the two main treatments
for varicose veins. Support hose squeeze your legs and prevent
blood from pooling in the veins. Exercise also helps keep blood
from pooling. When your leg muscles contract, they squeeze nearby
veins and help pump blood back to the heart. Surgery is reserved for
very severe cases of varicose veins.

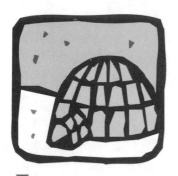

My feet are cold. Does this mean I have poor circulation? How can I warm them?

▼

TIP:

Many things can cause cold feet. It may be a sign of poor circulation, but it is not a reliable sign. If you think you have poor circulation, have your feet evaluated by your health care provider.

The best thing to do for cold feet is to wear one or two pairs of thick socks or warm house slippers. You can try the thin silk socks that are worn under regular socks for added warmth—but check to be sure that your shoes are not too tight. Getting up and walking around or getting regular exercise helps keep your feet warmer, too.

Do not use heating pads or hot water bottles on your feet. Don't sit too close to a space heater, fireplace, or campfire. If you have any diabetic nerve damage, you cannot feel when your feet are too hot or are getting burned, and you could be badly injured.

In addition to making your feet feel cold, nerve damage can affect blood flow and sweating in the feet. People with these problems are not able to release heat from their feet by dilating blood vessels the way someone without nerve damage would. It's best to wear socks and move around from time to time.

*O*ne or both of my feet are red, blue, purple, or darker
than they used to be. What do these colors mean?

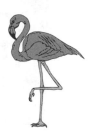

▼
TIP:

Changes in the color of the skin on your feet can mean many
things, from having gangrene to having the dye from your
socks rub off. Generally a color change alone does not tell you
enough to know whether it is caused by any specific disease.

Your health care provider will want to evaluate the color change
along with other signs and symptoms. She or he will look at your
skin, check the pulses in your thighs, ankles, and big toes, feel the
temperature of your skin, check for infections and broken bones,
and evaluate the blood circulation to your feet and legs.

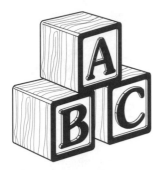

What is peripheral vascular disease?

▼
TIP:

Peripheral vascular disease (PVD) is commonly called "poor circulation" and refers to blockage in the blood supply to the feet. A buildup of plaque inside the artcries that carry blood to the feet causes them to thicken and harden. People without diabetes get this thickening and hardening of the arteries too, but unfortunately these problems can happen sooner and appear to be more severe in people with diabetes. PVD is 20 times more common in people with diabetes than in the general population. Other things that put you at risk of developing PVD are smoking, poor nutrition, lack of exercise, high blood fat levels (including cholesterol), and poor blood sugar control. Women are just as much at risk, and young as well as older people can develop it.

You can help to avoid or limit PVD by stopping smoking and controlling your blood fats levels and blood sugar levels as much as possible. See an RD for help with your meal plan and add more physical activity to your lifestyle.

*H*ow *does diabetes cause PVD?*

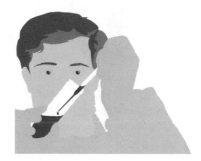

▼
TIP:

The fats in your blood, such as cholesterol and triglycerides, can build up on the walls of your arteries, thickening and hardening them. Diabetes often causes an increase in blood fats, which can lead to the thickening process. This is why your health care provider is concerned about checking your cholesterol and triglyceride levels, two important blood fats. If you have high cholesterol or high triglycerides, you may be asked to change your diet and to try to lose some weight. You may need to take medication to help control high cholesterol or high triglycerides.

It is important to control blood fats because the thickening of the arteries that leads to PVD can also cause heart attacks and strokes. You are at greater risk for these illnesses when you have diabetes.

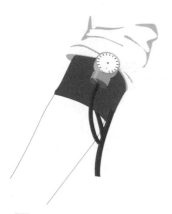

*W*hat kind of tests do I need for PVD?

▼
TIP:

Your health care provider will ask questions about your symptoms. He or she will examine your feet and legs and feel for foot and leg pulses, located in the groin, behind the knee, at the ankle, and on top of the foot. You may need to have the blood pressure in your ankle, arm, legs, and toes checked. (The arteries in toes don't get stiff, so measuring blood pressure there may be more accurate.) A doppler machine may be used, and this test is painless. You may need a test to measure how much oxygen gets to the skin of your feet. If you have an ulcer that won't heal or areas of your foot that break down despite wearing properly fitted shoes, you may need tests such as special X rays and scans. These tests give pictures of the blood flow from your thigh to your toes. For angiogram or arteriogram X rays, you get an intravenous injection of a special solution so the blood vessels show up clearly on the X ray. This solution is called "dye," although it really does not change the color of anything. To keep the dye from causing problems in your kidneys, your provider will give you intravenous fluids before and after the procedure. If you have questions, ask your provider and the people performing the tests to explain things to you.

*W*hat does smoking have to do with my feet?

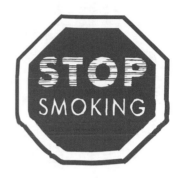

▼
TIP:

Smoking is clearly connected to developing vascular (heart and blood vessel) disease. When you smoke, the combustion products of tobacco are absorbed in the bloodstream. These chemicals stimulate the release of other chemicals, which injure the blood vessels and encourage thickening and hardening of the arteries. Smoking also causes your blood vessels to constrict or clamp down, which limits the amount of blood that can circulate.

Smoking and diabetes are a deadly combination for the vascular system. Fortunately, there are many new medications and good programs to help people quit smoking. If you smoke and you're ready to quit, ask your health care provider to refer you to one of these programs to help you do it.

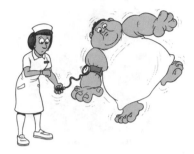

*W*hat does high blood pressure have to do with my feet?

▼
TIP:

High blood pressure (hypertension) damages the blood vessels all over your body and is associated with developing poor circulation. High blood pressure is most related to heart attacks, strokes, and kidney disease, but it also contributes to PVD. If you have diabetes, you need to try to control your blood pressure as well as you can. We know that 35–75% of all diabetic complications result from a combination of high blood pressure and diabetes.

You can help control your blood pressure by changing your meal plan and introducing more physical activity into your lifestyle.

*A*re there any treatments for PVD?

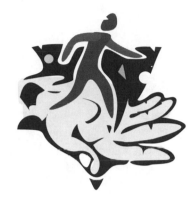

▼
TIP:

P reventing vascular disease is much easier than treating it. That is why your health care provider will stress that you quit smoking, control blood pressure and blood sugar, control cholesterol and triglycerides, lose weight, and stay active. Taking an aspirin a day can help prevent heart attacks and strokes, so some people think this might help prevent PVD, too. Aspirin is not recommended for every-one and can interact with other medications you may be taking, so ask your provider before you start taking aspirin daily.

There are some medications your doctor can prescribe to treat PVD. If you have intermittent claudication (pain in your calves with walking), you might be asked to walk more. Usually you are encouraged to walk to the point of pain, pause, and then walk a little more. Ask your provider to give you instructions. Walking may help stimulate new vessels to grow and this will improve circulation.

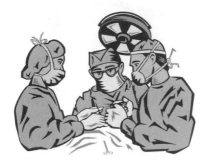

*W*ill *I need surgery for PVD?*

▼
TIP:

If the tests for PVD show that you have blockage in the larger arteries to your feet or legs, surgeons may try to correct it. One surgery that is not often used for patients with diabetes cleans out the artery that is blocked. Another method called angioplasty involves passing a deflated balloon on a tube to the point where the blockage occurs. Then the balloon is carefully inflated to open the narrowed artery and sometimes a stent (a tiny metal device shaped like a spring) is inserted in the artery to keep it open. This surgery is most successful with a small blockage in a healthy artery. A third surgical method is to bypass the blocked area by using a blood vessel from another part of the body (or an artificial blood vessel). While complicated, this surgery can help save a foot. People with diabetes often have many blockages in the arteries of the lower legs and feet, making it difficult to restore circulation. The relatively new ability to do bypass surgery down to the small arteries of the foot has saved many legs. Not all vascular surgeons do this surgery, so check to be sure that yours can. Your providers will carefully evaluate your condition before recommending surgery. If you must have surgery for PVD, ask your doctors to explain the procedure to you.

Chapter 10
OTHER FOOT PROBLEMS

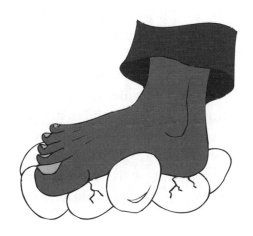

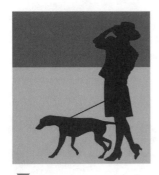

I have arthritis in my foot. How is this going to react with diabetes?

▼
TIP:

Arthritis is a general term that refers to wear and tear on the joints. There are different kinds of arthritis and different treatments for each kind. It is best to let your health care provider diagnose and treat any problems you are having with your joints. Don't assume that any pain, swelling, or stiffness in your foot is "just arthritis." There are many over-the-counter medications for treating arthritis, but consult your health care provider if you take these regularly.

Since both arthritis and diabetes tend to affect us as we get older, it is common to have both conditions. Arthritis can make it difficult for people with diabetes to stay as active as they need to be. However, because exercising and staying active are treatments for both arthritis and diabetes, you get a double dose of benefits whenever you exercise.

There are many new medications for arthritis. The current thinking is that arthritis should be treated more aggressively than it was in years past. Researchers think that starting treatment early could prevent much of the pain and disability associated with arthritis.

Arthritis can limit motion in the big toe joint, which can cause a callus or an ulcer under the big toe.

I have gout in my foot. How is this going to react with diabetes?

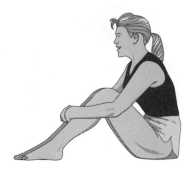

▼
TIP:

Gout is a special type of arthritis caused by an excess of uric acid in the blood. Uric acid crystals tend to settle in joints in the lowest part of the body, which is why the big toe is most often affected. These crystals can cause the big toe joint to become extremely painful, red, warm, and swollen. If you have the symptoms of gout, your health care provider may withdraw some joint fluid and examine it under a microscope to look for these crystals. Medications and a special diet to lower the uric acid levels in the body are the main treatments for gout.

Sometimes it is difficult to tell the difference between gout and an infection caused by bacteria. So, if you think you might have gout, it is important to see your health care provider.

Repeated episodes of gout tend to damage the big toe joint and may make it stiff. This can cause a high-pressure spot on your foot that is more prone to developing callus and an ulcer. Be sure to check your feet daily for any signs of redness or ulceration.

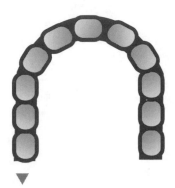

*W*hat is Charcot's joint and how do I recognize it?

▼
TIP:

Charcot's joint or Charcot foot is the term used to describe a severe deformity in a weight-bearing joint. A French physician named J. M. Charcot first described it in the 1860s. Charcot foot refers to the breakdown of the arch and normal foot structure in a person with nerve damage. Because Charcot's joint usually happens to people who have nerve damage, there is not much pain, even though they may have broken bones. There may be redness, swelling, and increased warmth of the foot. Your shoes won't fit. That's when people usually go to see their provider. Stay off that foot. The breakdown may occur fairly quickly. Sometimes it is difficult even for experts to tell the difference between Charcot's joint and infection.

Treatments for Charcot's joint are to immobilize the foot in a cast or special boot and rest the foot so it can heal. Sometimes surgery is done to realign the joints of the foot. If you continue to walk on a foot with Charcot's joint, you will make it much worse. If you can't get your regular shoes on, or if you have any changes in foot shape along with redness, swelling, or warmth, report this immediately to your health care provider.

W hat is osteomyelitis and how do I recognize it?

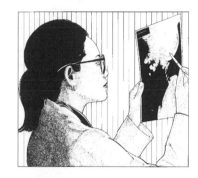

▼
TIP:

O steomyelitis is the medical name for an infection in the bone. If you have a foot ulcer that is not healing well, your health care provider will want to examine your foot with an X ray or scan to determine whether the nearby bones have been affected. This is important because the treatments for bone infection and for soft tissue infection are different. It is also extremely difficult to heal foot ulcers over infected bone. Sometimes surgery is required to remove bone infections.

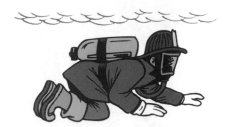

W *hat is gangrene?*
What causes it?

▼
TIP:

G angrene is a term that refers to death of the skin and the underlying tissues. The area of gangrene usually becomes dark brown or black. Once the tissue is dead, it will not grow back.

Severe circulation problems or infection can cause gangrene. Sometimes when a small toe becomes gangrenous, it may be left to just dry up and fall off. Other times the gangrene may be spreading and may need to be removed by surgery. You may need bypass surgery to improve circulation, which will help stop the gangrene from spreading, preserve as much of the toe or foot as possible, and prevent further problems.

I *had to have a toe amputation. Am I*
doomed?

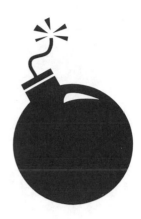

▼
TIP:

No, you are not doomed! However, once you have an amputation, you are at much higher risk for having another one. That is why you need to do everything you can to prevent diabetic foot problems. Check your feet daily, have your provider check your feet at every visit, and try to keep your blood fats and blood sugar levels as close to normal as possible. An amputation can "create" a foot deformity and put unusual pressure on the bones in your foot. You'll need orthotics, padding, or special shoes to be sure that you don't cause another ulcer on this foot. You might need physical therapy to learn how to walk smoothly. You would probably benefit from counseling or joining a support group of other people who have had amputations. You are likely to feel some pretty strong emotions after an experience like this.

Many people who have had a toe, foot, or leg amputation lead full and active lives. Medical science has made excellent breakthroughs in artificial limbs and rehabilitation for people with amputations.

Chapter 11
RESOURCES

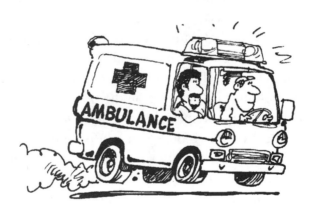

American Academy of
  Orthopaedic Surgeons
6300 North River Road
Rosemont, IL 60018-4262
(847) 823-7186
(800) 346-AAOS
website: *www.aaos.org*

American Association of
  Diabetes Educators
444 North Michigan Avenue,
  Suite 1240
Chicago, IL 60611
(312) 644-2233
(800) 832-6874

American Board of
  Podiatric Surgery
3330 Mission Street
San Francisco, CA 94110
(415) 826-3200
website: *www.abps.org*

American College of Foot and
  Ankle Surgeons
515 Busse Highway
Park Ridge, IL 60068
(847) 292-2237
(800) 421-2237
email: *mail@acfas.org*
website: *www.acfas.org*

American Diabetes Association
1701 North Beauregard Street
Alexandria, VA 22311
(703) 549-1500
(800) DIABETES
website: *www.diabetes.org*
bookstore: *www.store.diabetes.org*

American Orthopaedic Foot and
  Ankle Society
1216 Pine Street, Suite 201
Seattle, WA 98101-1944
(206) 223-1120
email: *aofas@aofas.org*
webpage: *http://www.aofas.org*

American Podiatric
  Medical Association
9312 Old Georgetown Road
Bethesda, MD 20814-1698
(301) 571-9200
(800) 275-2762
website: *www.apma.org*

Feet Can Last a Lifetime (video)
Available through:
Bureau of Primary Health Care
2070 Chain Bridge Road,
  Suite 450
Vienna, VA 22182
(703) 821-2098
Information kit with video: $15

International Diabetic Athletes
Association
1647 W. Bethany Home Road, #B
Phoenix, AZ 85015
(800) 898-IDAA
email: *idaa@getnet.com*
website: *http://www.getnet.com/
  ~idaa*

Lower Extremity Amputation
  Prevention Program (LEAP)
Bureau of Primary Health Care
  (BPHC)
Division of Programs for
  Special Populations
4350 East West Highway,
  9th Floor
Bethesda, MD 20814
(301) 594-4424
website: *bphc.hrsa.dhhs.gov/leap/*

National Chronic Pain
  Outreach Association
P.O. Box 274
Millboro, VA 24460
(540) 997-5004
email: *ncpoa1@aol.com*

National Odd Shoe Exchange
7102 North 35th Avenue, Suite 2
Phoenix, AZ 85051
(602) 841-6691

Neuropathy Association
60 E. 42nd Street, Suite 942
New York, NY 10165
(800) 247-6968
website: *www.neuropathy.org*

Pedorthic Footwear Association
9861 Broken Land Parkway,
  Suite 255
Columbia, MD 21046-1151
(800) 673-8447

President's Council on Physical
  Fitness and Sports
701 Pennsylvania Avenue, NW,
  Suite 250
Washington, DC 20004
(202) 272-3421

State-based Diabetes Control
  Programs funded by the Centers
  for Disease Control (CDC)
CDC Division of Diabetes
  Translation
P.O. Box 8728
Silver Spring, MD 20910
(877) 232-3422
email: *diabetes@cdc.gov*

INDEX

Blood glucose, *see* Blood sugar.
Blood pressure, 28–29, 100, 103
Blood sugar levels, 4, 5, 7, 10, 18, 25, 36, 59, 66, 69, 76, 79–81, 83, 86, 98, 103, 111
Blood vessels, 11, 28, 69, 101, 104
Blood vessel damage, 2, 10, 98, 101, 104
Brace, 91
Bunions, 3, 8, 12, 40, 66
Bypass surgery, 104, 110

C
Calf, 94
Callus, 3, 8, 12, 13, 15, 17, 40, 49, 51–52, 54, 61, 64–65, 68, 72–73, 78, 106–107
Callus removers, 62
Campfire, 96
Cane, 17, 91
Capsaicin creams, 83–84
Car, 28
Carpeting, 41
Certified diabetes educator (CDE), 11
Charcot's joint, 9, 78, 108
Chlorine bleach, 25
Cholesterol, 98–99
Circulation, *see* Blood circulation.
Cold feet, 94, 96
Color, 94
Complications, 2, 5, 6, 7, 10
Corn removers, 62
Corns, 3, 8, 13, 15, 17, 51, 61, 63
Cotton balls, 25
Counseling, 111
Crutches, 74
Custom-made shoes, 42, 47–48, 54, 111

D
Debride (dead tissue), 74
Deformity, 13, 40, 42, 47, 49, 52–54, 61, 68, 78, 81, 108, 111
Diabetes Control and Complications Trial (DCCT), 10
Diabetes educator, 11
Diabetic bullae, 57
Diuretics, 29
Doppler machine, 100
Drysol, 88

Dye, 100

E
Emery board, 32, 64
Erectile dysfunction, 81
Evening primrose oil, 83
Exercise, 7, 17, 18, 68–70, 89, 95–96, 98, 106

F
Fainting, 80
Fever, 25, 76
Fireplace, 96
Fitting shoes, 11, 42, 45, 54
Flexibility, 16
Food, 7
Foot bath, 20, 21
Foot color, 94, 97, 110
Foot odor, 27, 49
Foot swelling, 28–30
Foot surgery, 11, 12
Footwear, 9, 12, 41–45, 53
Fruits, 18
Fungus, 4, 18, 36, 60, 88

G
Gait, 9, 17, 52, 91
Gangrene, 110
Gastroparesis, 81
Germs, 4, 21, 26, 56
Glasses, 15
Green clay poultice, 62, 64
Gout, 107

H
Hair growth, 94
Hammertoes, 8, 12, 40, 61, 81
Health care providers, 11, 14, 17, 22, 23, 24, 27, 36, 37, 47, 57, 64, 66, 73–76, 83, 100–101, 104, 106
Heart, 28–29, 81, 101
Heart attacks, 99, 102–103
Heating pads, 96
High blood pressure, 28, 50, 102
High blood sugar, 4, 59, 73, 76, 79, 83
High pressure areas, 49, 64, 72, 107
Hispanic Americans, 5

R

Registered dietitian (RD), 18, 98
Risk factors, 6, 9, 21, 98
Rowing, 69
Running, 68
Running shoes, 8–9, 40, 68, 70

S

Sandals, 26, 68
Scans, 100
Senior centers, 15, 32
Sensory nerves, 78, 81, 90
Sexual functioning, 80
Skin, 4, 8, 13, 22, 24, 72, 78, 84, 88–89, 97
Skin oils, 21, 22
Shoehorn, 16
Shoes, 8, 9, 14, 17, 26, 27, 40, 42–45, 56–57, 63–64, 70, 73, 86, 88, 100
Shower, 20
Smoking, 98, 101, 103
Soaking, 21, 73
Soap, 20, 22
Sock puller, 16
Socks, 8, 14, 23, 26, 27, 30, 46, 56–57, 68, 73, 86, 88, 96–97
Sores, 13
Space heater, 96
Sponges, 16
Stair climbers, 68
Stomach, 81
Stretching, 16, 68–69, 83
Strokes, 99, 102–103
Sulfonylureas, 83
Support hose, 30, 95
Surgery, 8, 32, 58, 61, 63–66, 75, 94, 104, 108–110
Sweating, 22, 78, 81, 88–89, 96
Swelling, 28–29, 50, 58, 106–108
Swimming, 26, 68–69

T

Temperature, checking, 20, 97
Tests, 82, 97, 100
Tetanus, 59
Thyroid disease, 82

Toenails, 8, 15, 32(38, 60
Towels, 20, 26
Triglycerides, 99, 103
Tuning fork, 13, 80, 82
Type 1 diabetes, 6, 10
Type 2 diabetes, 6, 10

U

Ulcer, 2, 3, 5, 9, 11, 27, 36, 40, 42, 47, 49(50, 68, 72(76, 94, 100, 106(107, 109, 111
Unexplained high blood sugar, 59, 76
United Kingdom Prospective Diabetes Study (UKPDS), 10
Upper body exercises, 69
Uric acid, 107

V

Varicose veins, 95
Vascular surgeons, 11, 75
Vascular surgery, 94
Vegetable oils, 23
Vegetables, 18
Veins, 95
Vision problems, 15, 32
Vitamin deficiencies, 82
Vomiting, 80

W

Walking, 68(69, 90(91, 94(96, 103
Warning signs, 13
Wart, 65
Water, 68
Water pills, 29
Weight, 9, 99, 103
Weight lifting, 69
Wheel chair, 74
Wool, 23
Wounds, 13, 21, 27, 56, 72, 74, 76, 84

X

X ray, 58, 100, 109

Y

Yoga, 16, 69

About the American Diabetes Association

The American Diabetes Association is the nation's leading voluntary health organization supporting diabetes research, information, and advocacy. Founded in 1940, the Association provides services to communities across the country. Its mission is to prevent and cure diabetes and to improve the lives of all people affected by diabetes.

For more than 50 years, the American Diabetes Association has been the leading publisher of comprehensive diabetes information for people with diabetes and the health care professionals who treat them. Its huge library of practical and authoritative books for people with diabetes covers every aspect of self-care—cooking and nutrition, fitness, weight control, medications, complications, emotional issues, and general self-care. The Association also publishes books and medical treatment guides for physicians and other health care professionals.

Membership in the Association is available to health care professionals and people with diabetes and includes subscriptions to one or more of the Association's periodicals. People with diabetes receive *Diabetes Forecast*, the nation's leading health and wellness magazine for people with diabetes. Health care professionals receive one or more of the Association's five scientific and medical journals.

For more information, please call toll-free:

Questions about diabetes:	1-800-DIABETES
Membership, people with diabetes:	1-800-806-7801
Membership, health professionals:	1-800-232-3472
To order ADA books or receive a free catalog:	1-800-232-6733
Visit us on the Web:	www.diabetes.org
Visit us at our Web bookstore:	store.diabetes.org